BodyTalk

BodyTalk

365 GENTLE MOVEMENT PRACTICES to GET OUT of YOUR HEAD and INTO YOUR BODY

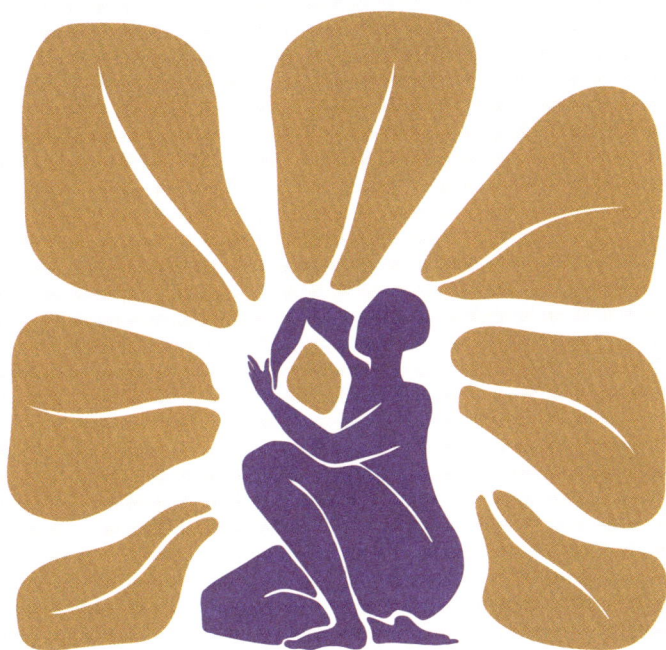

Erica Hornthal,
LCPC, BC-DMT

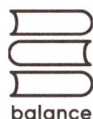

balance

New York   Boston

Copyright © 2025 by Erica Hornthal
Cover design by Jim Datz
Cover image by Shutterstock
Cover copyright © 2025 by Hachette Book Group, Inc.

Balance
Hachette Book Group
1290 Avenue of the Americas
New York, NY 10104
GCP-Balance.com
@GCPBalance

First Edition: July 2025

Balance is an imprint of Grand Central Publishing. The Balance name and logo are registered trademarks of Hachette Book Group, Inc.

The publisher is not responsible for websites (or their content) that are not owned by the publisher.

The Hachette Speakers Bureau provides a wide range of authors for speaking events. To find out more, go to hachettespeakersbureau.com or email HachetteSpeakers@hbgusa.com.

Balance books may be purchased in bulk for business, educational, or promotional use. For information, please contact your local bookseller or the Hachette Book Group Special Markets Department at special.markets@hbgusa.com.

Print book interior design by Amy Quinn.

Library of Congress Cataloging-in-Publication Data

Names: Hornthal, Erica, 1983– author.
Title: Body talk : 365 gentle movement practices to get out of your head and into your body / Erica Hornthal, LCPC, BC-DMT.
Description: First edition. | New York : Balance, [2025] | Includes bibliographical references.
Identifiers: LCCN 2024062119 | ISBN 9781538771525 (trade paperback) | ISBN 9781538771532 (ebook)
Subjects: LCSH: Mind and body. | Movement, Psychology of.
Classification: LCC BF161 .H768 2025 | DDC 128/.2—dc23/eng/20250319
LC record available at https://lccn.loc.gov/2024062119

ISBNs: 9781538771525 (trade paperback), 9781538771532 (ebook)

Printed in the United States of America

VER

10 9 8 7 6 5 4 3 2 1

This book is dedicated to the bodies that are scared, lost, insecure, invisible, traumatized, and isolated. The bodies that are bracing, holding it together, pushing through, floundering, and surviving. The bodies in need of connection. The bodies that are talking when no one is listening. I see you. I hear you. Welcome home.

Contents

Introduction

A S A CHILD, MY MIND HOUSED THE IMAGINARY FRIENDS THAT understood me, the worries that kept me safe and in control of my uncontrollable environment, the witty banter that kept me entertained, and the ability to overanalyze everything. As I got older, my mind also housed the judgment, criticism, and negative self-talk that convinced me I wasn't enough—not smart enough, not pretty enough, not perfect enough, not good enough.

Thanks to an educational system and a society that prioritize verbal communication and intellect over felt experience and sensory processing, I learned to live "in my head," as many of us do, separated from my felt experience, senses, and body altogether. Now, with the proliferation of handheld devices such as tablets and phones, we are a society of heads carried by bodies that are valued more for how they look and how much they can do and less for what they feel and how they simply exist. I have been a dancer for most of my life, but that still did not teach me to appreciate and listen to my body but rather to allow it to be ridiculed by my mind and conditioned into unrealistic standards of beauty, performance, and achievement.

It wasn't until I ventured into the field of dance/movement therapy that I began to uncover my own fear around, insecurity about, and lack of awareness of my own body. I became aware of how disconnected I was from my own felt experiences as a dancer but also realized that dance was in many ways what allowed me to keep moving through life. So many of us are wandering through this life insecure, detached, disconnected, and anxious. It's actually gotten to the point that not only do we *not* know how we feel, but we also do not know how to *connect* to what we feel.

You are here because you recognize that you've lost that ability to connect to what you feel. Whether this severed connection is the result of chronic stress, trauma, injury, illness, or a congenital condition, you deserve to reestablish a synergy between your mind and your body. You deserve to live a life beyond the confines of your mind. You do not need to understand what you feel in order to heal.

Establishing a secure connection to our emotions begins with establishing a secure connection to our body, where the emotions are housed. Like a muscle that has been neglected, the connection to our body atrophies over time if not exercised, and to establish safety with the unknown and unfamiliar, we must slowly reorient and reintroduce felt experiences with gentle curiosity and compassion.

For many of us who have experienced trauma, the body can be a scary place. You may have found your way to this book because you are looking for support in response to years of chronic pain or illness, injury, or a degenerative or cognitive ailment. Regardless of the reason, connecting to your felt experience can feel like returning to the scene of a crime. Getting back in sync with your body doesn't automatically bring comfort and peace. It is a gradual process, one that may turn over some fear and uncertainty. It's not as simple as trying on a somatic exercise or engaging in a somatic workout. This work requires validation and witnessing along the way.

Healing happens in a relationship, and that begins with the one we have with our own body. This journal is your first step toward reestablishing a symbiotic and harmonious relationship with your body as a way to support your physical and emotional well-being, to live the life you deserve, and to manage human emotions rather than react to them. Learning to listen and understand what your body is saying without judgment and without the need to fix it is a powerful method for managing mental health and riding the waves of life.

A healthy mind begins with the ability to converse with your body. When we are born into existence, we sense everything. Over time as our mind develops, we rely more on thinking and reasoning and become less reliant, comfortable, and trusting of what we feel and sense in our body. *BodyTalk* is a guide to learning the language of your individual body. Over the next 365 days, you'll embark on a journey to reconnect to your body and felt sensations. Engaging in this journey is about reclaiming and repatterning much of your association with movement to reestablish a secure connection to your felt experiences without overwhelming your nervous system or perpetuating stress or trauma.

HOW TO USE THIS BOOK

THIS BOOK IS SPLIT INTO TWELVE SECTIONS, EACH BUILDING ON THE previous one. It provides fundamental experiences that create the foundation for psychological development through movement. Revisiting these experiences is vital for developing a healthy connection between mind and body. You can revisit or focus on any section that feels relevant to you. The most important "rule" for this book is to take your time. Part of reconnecting to the body is about noticing the tendency to rush through, overwhelm, and take on too much, which only serve to perpetuate our inability to connect to the present moment. You can use this book when you need a break, feel overwhelmed, or need a reminder to drop back into your body to find respite from your mind. It can become a 365-day practice or ritual that supports a healthy connection to and dialogue with your body. You can begin and end your day with the daily exercise or revisit the exercise throughout the day if you so choose.

Feel free to integrate journaling, creative art making, movement, and music into your experience as well. Including elements that support your growth and curiosity as you reengage with your body is crucial to building trust and ease as you go.

Some of the prompts and activities may appear simple, but their cumulative effect over the course of the year will yield great results. Keep in mind that, although many of these prompts can be adapted to your individual needs, only you know what it feels like to be in your body. Proceed with all exercises using caution and compassion for your body's individual needs and abilities.

Give yourself permission to step away when needed. This may be a daily guide, but there is no prize for completion. The rewards you seek are a relationship with your inner and outer experience and freedom from the cage that has become your mind.

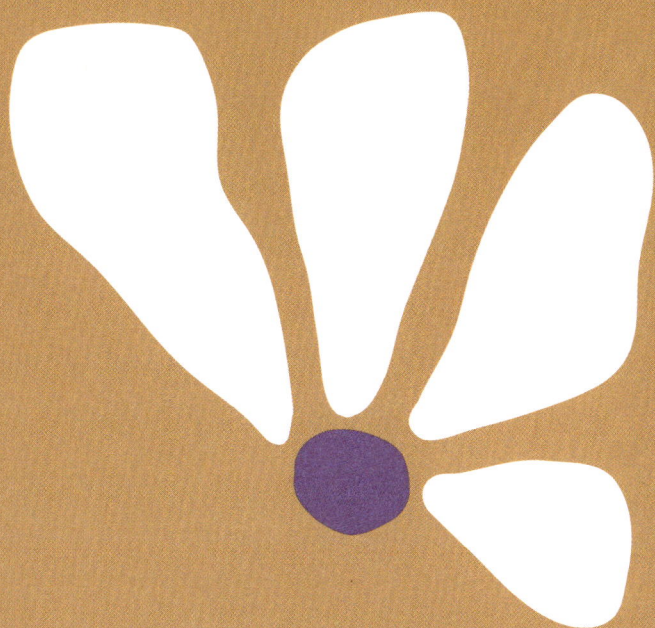

FOUNDATIONS

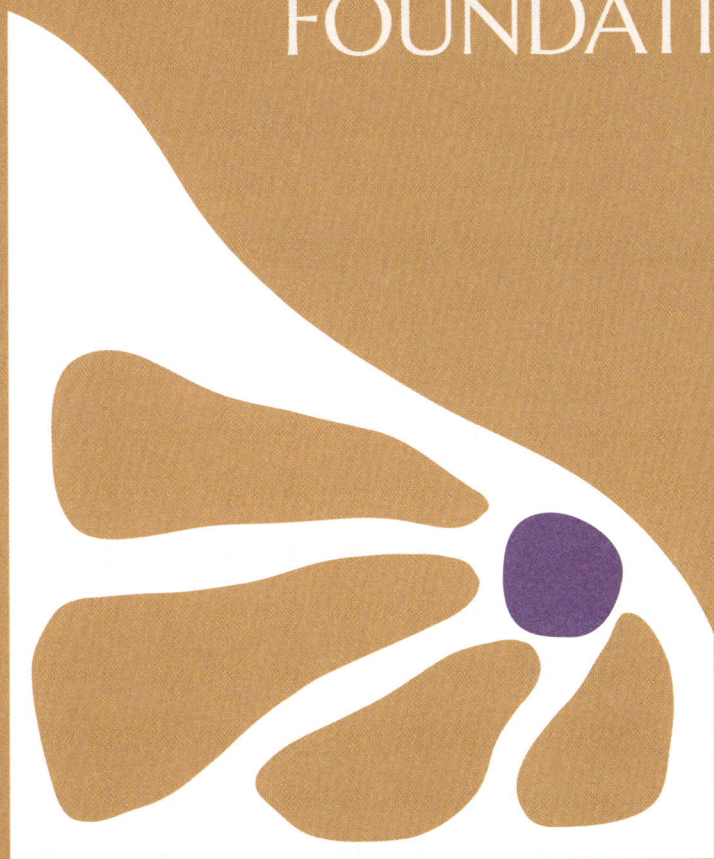

The body holds answers to questions the mind doesn't even know to ask.

DAY 1
How Are You *Moving* Today?

TAKE A MOMENT TO NOTICE ALL THE MOVEMENT THAT IS PRESENT and all the movement that is absent. Some examples are breathing, blinking, sitting, and walking. Consider the qualities of your movement as well, such as *heavy*, *light*, *quick*, or *slow*. Be as specific as possible. As insignificant as a movement might seem, it could be the difference between autopilot and awareness.

"How are you *moving* today?" is an important question, and one we'll revisit throughout this journey. Any moment is an opportunity to change how we feel by becoming more aware of how we are moving.

Document this exploration in any way that works for you—write it down, either in the space provided here or in your journal or notes app, or create art or music that expresses where you are on this journey. This will serve as a reminder and baseline as you continue to check in throughout the year.

....

....

....

....

....

....

....

....

....

....

....

....

DAY 2
Set Intentions

CREATE A LIST OF INTENTIONS YOU HAVE FOR ENGAGING WITH THIS book. What are you hoping to gain from this daily journey? Identify intentions for your mind—for example, *Slow down my anxious thoughts* and *Reduce negative self-talk*—and intentions for your body, such as *Relax my shoulders, find stillness in my body.*

....

....

....

....

....

....

....

....

....

....

....

....

....

....

....

....

....

....

DAY 3
What *Moves* You?

EVERY DAY WE ARE MOVED BY AND FOR PEOPLE, PLACES, AND CIR-cumstances. Make a list of the ways you move your body physically. It could be an exercise regimen, physical activities, hobbies, or even occupations. Take time to answer the following questions:

What is my current relationship to movement?
What are my preferred movement practices?
What movements do I prefer to stay away from?
When I move more, I feel . . .
When I move less, I feel . . .

Now, make a list of the things that move you emotionally. What makes you angry or excited? What moves you to tears?

....
....
....
....
....
....
....
....
....
....
....
....

DAY 4
What Influences Your Movement?

MAKE A LIST OF WHAT LIMITS YOU FROM MOVING, SUCH AS SPACE, time, injuries, or cognitive and physical differences.

....
....
....
....
....
....
....
....
....
....
....
....
....
....
....
....
....
....

DAY 5
Movement Fears

TAKE A FEW MINUTES TO JOURNAL ON WHAT FEARS YOU HAVE around movement. Some questions to consider are these:

What prevents me from moving?
If I move, I might . . .
If I stop moving, then I will . . .

....

....

....

....

....

....

....

....

....

....

....

....

....

....

....

....

....

DAY 6
Movement Myths

IDENTIFY MYTHS OR ASSUMED TRUTHS YOU HOLD ABOUT MOVEMENT.
For example, "All movement is exercise" or "No pain, no gain."

Where did I learn these?

....
....
....

Who else in my family holds these myths to be truths?

....
....
....

What do I notice when I challenge these myths or
question their validity?

....
....
....

DAY 7
Hide-and-Seek

CONSIDER THE PARTS OF YOUR BODY THAT YOU SHOW OFF AND THE parts that you hide. What are the stories you hold about these parts? Why do you hold them?

....

....

....

....

....

....

....

....

....

....

DAY 8
Don't Judge a Body by Its Cover

WHAT JUDGMENTS DO YOU MAKE ABOUT MOVEMENT? ARE SOME movements better than others? What movements do you see as good or bad?

Do you feel judged by others when you move your body? What critiques or praise have you heard from others about your movement or body?

....

....

....

....

....

....

....

....

....

....

....

....

....

....

....

....

....

....

DAY 9
Mind Your Body

THINK ABOUT THE WORD *BODY*. JOURNAL ABOUT WHAT THE WORD *body* means to you. Notice how you physically respond to this word. Before you can establish a connection to your body, it is important to understand the preconceived judgments being made about it. Connecting to your body requires a nonjudgmental, unbiased space in which it can be seen, acknowledged, and heard, first and foremost by you.

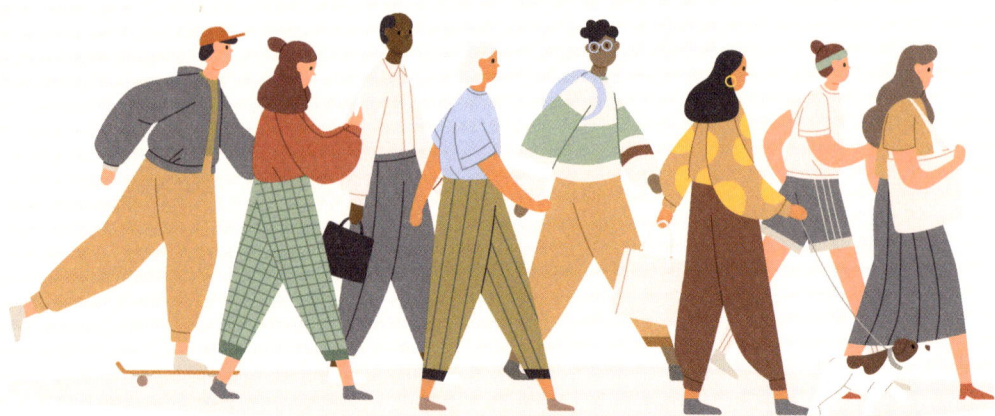

DAY 10
Witness Other Bodies

TAKE AT LEAST FIVE MINUTES TODAY TO WITNESS OTHER PEOPLE'S bodies and movements. Notice how quick you may be to judge those bodies. Do you notice any sensations or movements in your own body as you witness others in theirs?

Our bodies mirror the bodies around us. Notice how you move in relationship to those around you.

DAY 11
Be Moved

YOUR MOVEMENT IS INFLUENCED BY YOUR ENVIRONMENT. BECOME aware of your surroundings and allow them to move you.

Some examples may be walking around someone coming near you, following a curious sound, swaying with the breeze.

Whatever feels accessible to you in this moment, find a way to be moved physically by your environment.

DAY 12
Shift Happens

CHANGE CAN BE SEEN AS A SHIFT. WHEN LOOKING TO CHANGE HOW you relate to your body, you can invite in small shifts. Shift your body posture. Notice how shifting your body influences your mind. Any change in your movement is an opportunity to shift your mental perspective.

....

....

....

....

....

....

....

....

DAY 13
Find Comfort

TAKE THIS MOMENT TO BRING MORE COMFORT TO YOUR BODY. THIS may be through posture, temperature, or environment. Perhaps you are aware of the discomfort in your body. Use this as an invitation to ease your way into less discomfort.

....

....

....

....

....

....

....

DAY 14

Ease Your Discomfort

YOU MIGHT FIND THAT YOU AVOID, IGNORE, OR NUMB YOUR BODY TO ease your discomfort. Our brain is wired for comfort, so it makes sense we would want to avoid pain, suffering, or even the unfamiliar.

Try on an uncomfortable pose—but this should not cause physical pain. Then, ease your discomfort by repositioning your body into a more comfortable position.

Repeat this exercise two or three more times and notice how your relationship with the discomfort changes, as does the process of the overall transition.

DAY 15
Tracing

WITH YOUR INDEX FINGER OR HAND, BEGIN TRACING THE BORDERS of your body. Start at either end of your body and work your way up or down and then back again. After, take note of how you feel.

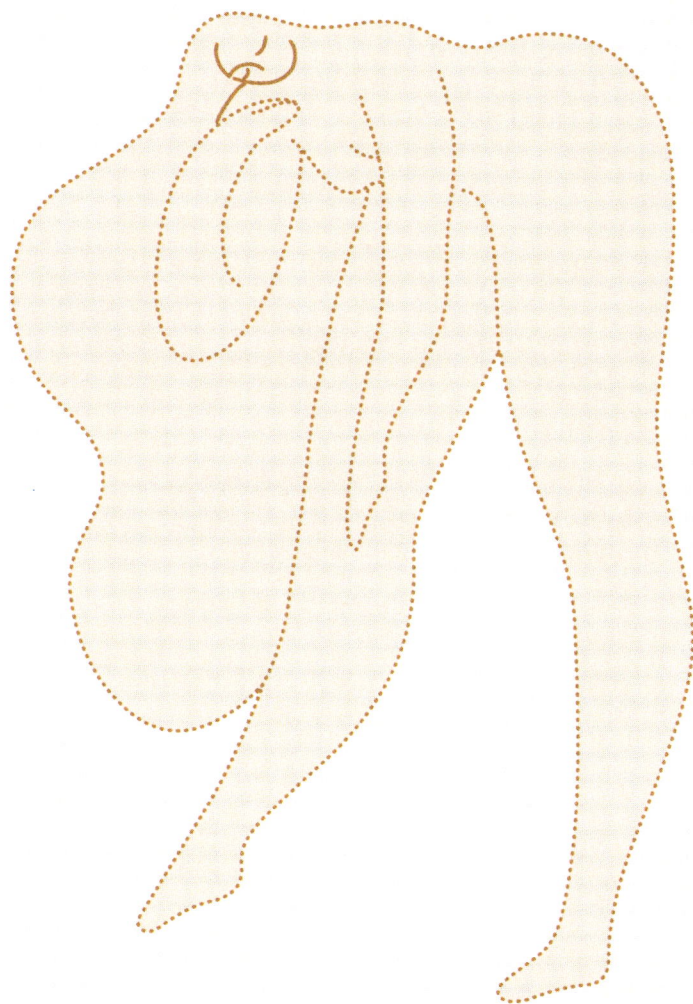

DAY 16
"I'm Touched!"

USING YOUR FINGERTIPS OR HANDS, TOUCH YOUR BODY. THIS CAN BE through light touch, massage, or a gentle squeeze. Touch is difficult for many of us. Safe touch begins with taking the opportunity to connect in a safe way to your body, recognizing what feels appropriate, nurturing, possible, and wanted.

DAY 17
Play with Texture

IDENTIFY A FEW DIFFERENT MATERIALS WITH DIFFERENT TEXTURES. Some examples might be a soft blanket, a coarse towel, an oily lotion, or a bristly hairbrush. Choose three or four available textures and allow them to touch your skin. Notice how each feels and identify which you prefer.

DAY 18
Distractions

TAKE INVENTORY OF WHAT PULLS AT YOUR ATTENTION.

What distractions are present that may prevent me from being in the moment, in my body, or connected to what I feel?

....

....

....

What distractions support disconnection from my body?

....

....

....

What happens in my mind and body when I think of the absence of these distractions?

....

....

....

DAY 19
Tune In

NOTICE WHAT YOU ARE AWARE OF IN THIS MOMENT. WHAT DO YOU feel around and inside your body? What parts do you find difficult to tune in to? Awareness of this is important as you continue to reconnect with your body.

....

....

....

....

....

....

....

....

....

....

DAY 20
Movement Mentors

HOW YOU SEE YOUR BODY HAS BEEN SHAPED BY THE BODIES THAT you were surrounded with growing up. Take a moment to identify who you learned your body narratives from. Who shaped your connection to or disconnection from your body?

....

....

....

....

....

....

....

....

....

....

DAY 21
Body Jobs

WHAT THINGS HAS YOUR BODY ALLOWED YOU TO DO? THIS COULD BE bearing children, expressing emotions, having intimate relations, experiencing pleasure, eating, or drinking.

Identify all the things your body is capable of that you might take for granted, such as breathing and digestion.

....

....

....

DAY 22

Anchor Yourself

WHEN REESTABLISHING A CONNECTION WITH YOUR BODY, IT IS important to maintain daily practices or rituals that connect you to your day. Identify two or three daily habits that are familiar, such as drinking a morning cup of coffee or walking a pet. These are important because they create an anchor, an action or sensory experience that generates reliability, stability, and support that serves to interrupt the status quo or autopilot.

....

....

....

DAY 23
Movement Preferences

HOW DO YOU PREFER TO MOVE YOUR BODY? WHAT MOVEMENT DOES it enjoy? What movement does it resist?

....

....

....

....

....

....

....

....

....

....

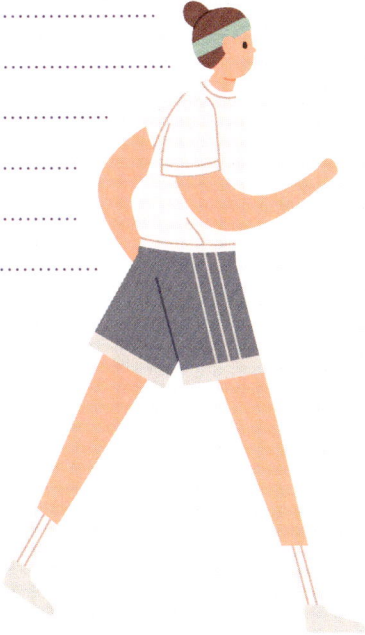

DAY 24
You Are How You Move

WHAT DOES YOUR CURRENT MOVEMENT SAY ABOUT YOU? DO YOU move in a way that supports the person you want to be?

....

....

....

....

....

....

....

....

....

....

DAY 25
Dressed to Move

CONSIDER THE IMPACT YOUR CLOTHING HAS ON YOUR MOVEMENT.
How might what you wear constrict your movement? Does what you
wear increase your ability to disconnect from your body?

....

....

....

....

....

....

....

....

....

....

....

DAY 26
Your Movement Signature

IDENTIFY YOUR MOVEMENT MANNERISMS AND GESTURES THAT YOU associate with individual self-expression or identity. What movements do you regularly engage in, such as adopting a certain posture, pose, or way of sitting or talking? Notice how you are sitting while engaging with this book. Don't change it. Just notice it.

....

....

....

....

....

....

....

....

....

....

....

DAY 27
Don't Be So Tense

PAY ATTENTION TO ANY TENSION PRESENT IN YOUR BODY. WHERE DO you typically carry your tension? (You may feel it in your shoulders, jaw, neck, head, or even your hips.)

....
....
....
....
....
....
....
....
....
....
....
....
....
....
....
....
....
....
....

DAY 28
Head, Shoulders, Knees, Toes

Using both hands, gently pat, squeeze, or rub your head, shoulders, knees, and toes consecutively. Now pay attention to what connects each of these parts. Slowly bring into your awareness how all these parts are connected.

DAY 29
Move Your Mind

If your mind were a person, how would it move? Without addressing the contents of your mind specifically, try moving in a way that expresses the rhythm, pace, and intensity of your thoughts.

DAY 30
How Are You *Moving?*

TAKE AN INVENTORY OF HOW YOU ARE MOVING IN THIS MOMENT.
What do you notice now compared with when you started on Day 1?

....
....
....
....
....
....
....
....
....
....
....
....
....
....
....
....
....
....
....

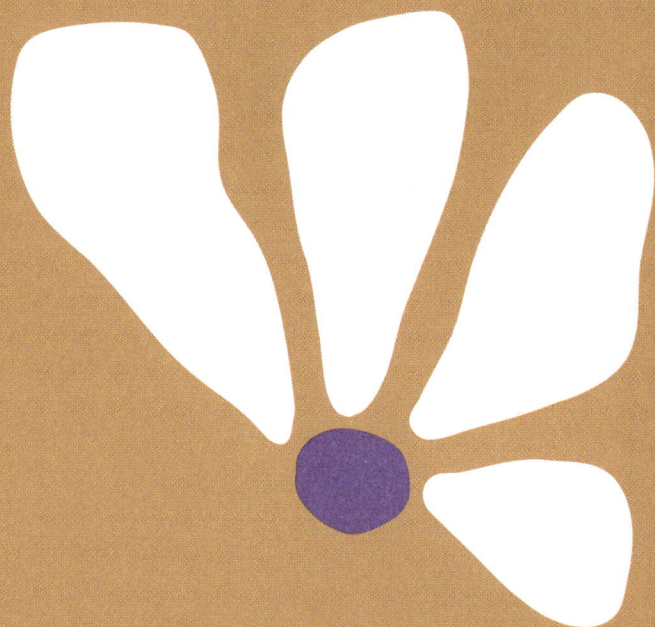

SENSATIONS

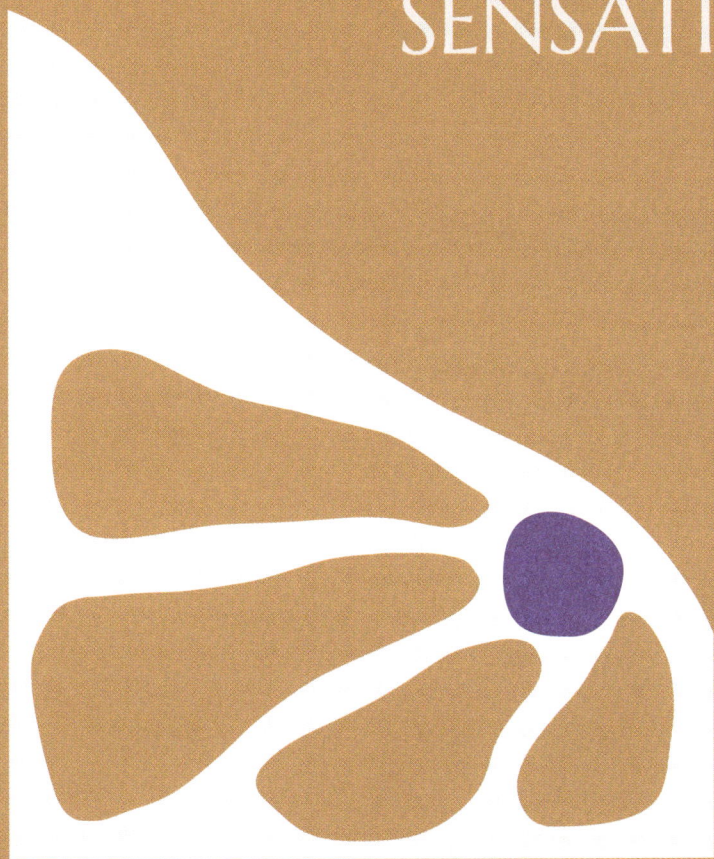

The mind communicates
through thought and judgment.

The body communicates
through sensation.

DAY 31
Five, Four, Three, Two, One . . .

LET'S PRACTICE AWARENESS OF THE SENSES. IDENTIFY THE following:

Five things you can see

Four things you can touch

Three things you can hear

Two things you can smell

One thing you can taste

You can use this practice to ground yourself in order to feel more connected to the present moment.

DAY 32
I See You

OPEN YOUR EYES AND SLOWLY LOOK AROUND. ALLOW YOUR EYES TO initiate the movement of your head rather than your head dictating what you focus your eyes on. Move with intentionality and steadiness. Let your sense of sight guide your movement.

DAY 33
Look Around

IN A VARIATION ON THE PREVIOUS PROMPT, TODAY YOU WILL FOCUS on moving your eyes while keeping your head stationary, ideally facing forward. Notice what is in your range of sight and what you can sense without the need to move your head. Become aware of your peripheral vision, how far you can see to each side while keeping your eyes looking straight ahead. Gently activate the muscles of your eyes by looking around and in all directions.

DAY 34
Focus

FOCUS ON A STATIONARY POINT IN FRONT OF YOU. ALLOW YOUR GAZE to soften. Now oscillate between focus and a soft gaze. Feel the difference between them. How does each vision state affect your internal and external awareness?

....
....
....
....
....
....
....
....
....
....
....
....
....
....
....
....
....
....

DAY 35
Make Contact

IDENTIFY AN OBJECT WITHIN EASY REACH. KEEPING YOUR EYES open, be mindful of the process of reaching for the object and touching it. Let your fingertips interact with the object before grasping it. Allow both hands to touch the object, manipulate it, and explore its textures.

DAY 36

Stop and Smell the . . .

IDENTIFY A SCENT THAT IS FAMILIAR AND INVITING. THIS MIGHT BE a perfume, a candle, a spice, or even a flower from your garden. Perhaps even a breath of fresh air from the outside. Pay attention to how your body feels as you invite the scent into your awareness.

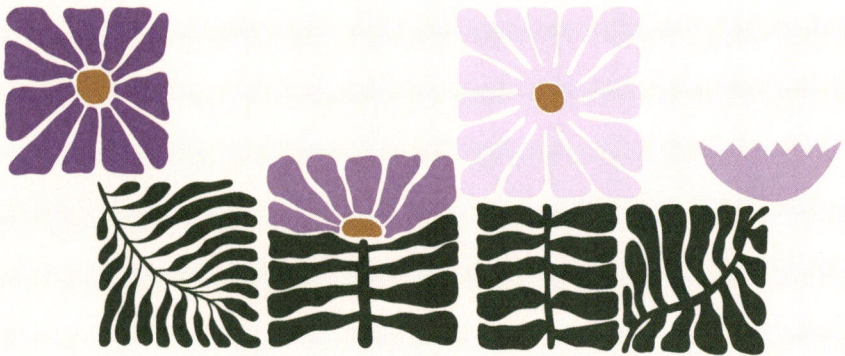

DAY 37
You Have Good Taste

CHOOSE A SMALL HARD CANDY, MINT, OR PIECE OF CHOCOLATE, IDEally of a taste you enjoy. Place the treat on your tongue and allow the flavor to take over your mouth. Let the food dissolve or melt entirely. Notice how this feels in your mouth as well as how the taste affects the rest of your body and mind.

DAY 38
I Hear You

BRING INTO YOUR AWARENESS ANY SOUNDS IN YOUR IMMEDIATE environment. Notice the need to identify what they are or where they are coming from and simply listen. Close your eyes and see how that changes your experience of the sounds. Pay attention to how your body reacts to or moves with the presence of the sounds.

DAY 39
Listen In

FOCUS ON A SOUND COMING FROM YOUR BODY. FOR EXAMPLE, THE breath entering or leaving your nose or mouth, your fingers rubbing together, a swallow, or perhaps the gurgling of your stomach. It may help to close your eyes to eliminate any visual stimulation. If nothing is audible to you in this moment, find a time throughout your day to listen in. This may be at mealtimes, during bathroom breaks, before falling asleep, or right after waking up.

DAY 40

Breathe in Awareness

NOTICE YOUR BREATH. THERE IS NO NEED TO CHANGE IT, BUT RATHER allow yourself to become aware of where you feel it. Take note of how deep or shallow it is in this moment.

DAY 41
Exploration in Space

Standing with your feet planted firmly on the ground or sitting with your bottom supported in a chair, explore the space around you. Allow your extremities to reach as far as possible without moving your feet from their current position. This is your *kinesphere*, your space bubble. Continue to explore as much of the space around you as you can while keeping your feet or bottom planted.

DAY 42
Locate Yourself

Identify an object within reach. With your eyes open, briefly touch or interact with the object. Now close your eyes and attempt to touch the object again. Were you able to find it right away? How long did it take for you to find the object with your eyes closed? This is an exercise in *proprioception*, your ability to perceive where you are in space. Sharpening your proprioceptive sense enhances your grounding.

....

....

....

....

....

....

....

DAY 43
Feeling Sole-ful

PLACE YOUR BARE FEET ON A FIRM SURFACE, SUCH AS A HARDWOOD or tiled floor. Imagine a triangle that connects your big toe, pinky toe, and heel of your foot. Feel your feet connect to the ground as you create even pressure across the sole of your foot.

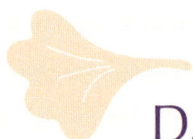

DAY 44
Earthing

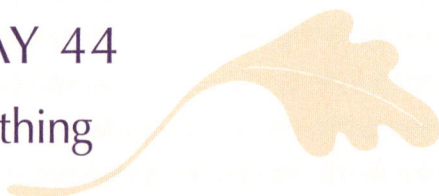

WITH BARE FEET, FIND A SECURE PATCH OF GRASS AND REPLICATE the previous day's exercise. Once connection is established, walk through the grass, feeling the earth underneath your feet. This practice allows for an exchange of energy, a reduction in electrical charge in the body, and a synchronization with the natural frequencies of Earth.

DAY 45
Gravity Takes Hold

BEGIN STANDING. LET YOUR BODY BE HEAVY. SLOWLY ALLOW GRAVity to pull you down to the ground. Find your way to a comfortable position lying down. With each breath cycle, allow your body to be held by the floor. Relinquish any tension present in your body.

DAY 46
Aw-Air-Ness

SITTING IN A CHAIR, BRING AWARENESS TO THE TEMPERATURE around your body. Can you feel the air as it touches your skin? Play with different temperatures to increase this awareness. For example, open the refrigerator and feel the cool air or step outside and notice the external temperature and how it feels on your skin.

....

....

....

....

....

....

....

....

....

....

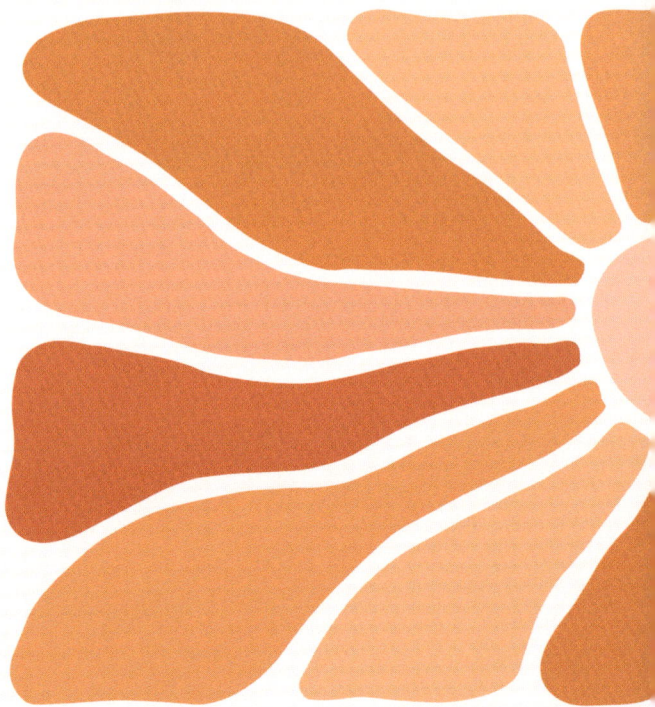

DAY 47
Warm Up

FEEL THE WARMTH OF THE SUN ON YOUR FACE. WITH CLOSED EYES, allow your chin to raise toward the sun. Stay here for a few minutes. Notice what changes you feel as the sun warms your face.

DAY 48
Wash Your Hands

BEGIN LATHERING YOUR HANDS WITH SOAP AND ROOM-TEMPERATURE water. As the lather builds, make contact with every nook and cranny of your hands and fingers. Be sure to lather each finger, nail bed, palm, and wrist. Mindfully wash your hands for twenty to thirty seconds. Become aware of the sensation and don't let it be simply the mundane task we usually do on autopilot.

DAY 49

Shower Yourself in Awareness

NEXT TIME YOU TAKE A SHOWER, PRACTICE BECOMING MORE AWARE of how the water feels as it runs down your body. Allow the water to guide you into a body scan as you connect to each part as the water runs down. Begin with the top of your head and feel the water run down each arm, the front and back of your body, and each leg. (You can do this in a bathing suit if it feels more comfortable to do so.)

DAY 50
Drink It In

GET A WARM OR COLD BEVERAGE.
Take a sip of the drink and become
aware of how it feels as it enters your
mouth and how it feels as you swallow. Take your time to be mindful
of the process. Replicate as many
times as you desire to increase the
awareness of this sensation.

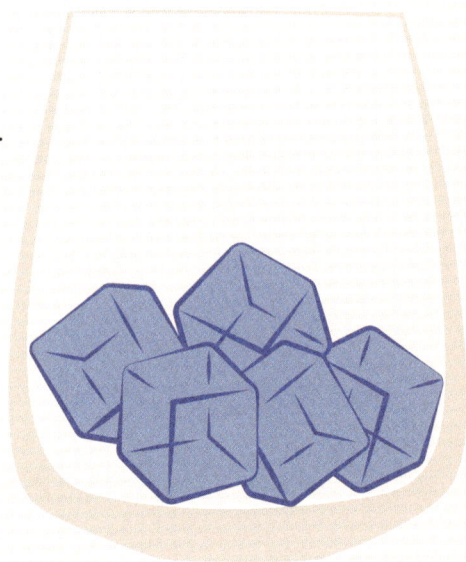

DAY 51
Trace Your Face

WITH YOUR INDEX FINGER, SLOWLY TRACE YOUR FACIAL FEATURES. Notice the texture of your skin and hair. Become aware of how your skin feels being touched by your finger and how your finger feels when touching your face. Feel the difference between your skin and your eyebrows or facial hair. Next, use several fingertips or the palm of your hand to cradle or caress your forehead and cheeks.

DAY 52
Hands Together

PRESS YOUR HANDS TOGETHER AS IN A PRAYER POSE. PLAY WITH DIFferent pressures as you push your palms and fingers together and then slowly pull them apart. Can you feel the difference between what your left hand feels and what your right hand feels?

DAY 53
Dressing Up

As you get dressed, pay attention to how each part of your body moves. Be mindful of each limb as the fabric touches it. Feel how your clothes rest on the surface of your skin. Bring your attention to the borders of each article of clothing. Can you feel the difference between the parts of your body that are covered with fabric and the parts that are bare?

....

....

....

....

....

....

....

....

....

....

....

....

....

....

....

....

DAY 54
Step Lightly

MOST OF US WALK ON AUTOPILOT, WITH VERY LITTLE AWARENESS OF how we are doing it. Draw your attention to your walk. Notice the sway of your hips and your gait, rhythm, and speed as you move through space. Notice how your feet make contact with the floor as they carry you forward.

DAY 55
Pet Something Soft

IF YOU OWN A PET OR FEEL COMFORTABLE PETTING SOMEONE ELSE'S animal, take a few minutes in your day to do so. If you do not have access to an animal, find a soft blanket or a stuffed animal. Allow your hand to make contact and slowly stroke the soft surface.

DAY 56
Tongue and Teeth

USING ONLY YOUR TONGUE, EXPLORE THE INSIDE OF YOUR MOUTH. You can count your teeth, glide your tongue across your gums, and explore the roof of your mouth.

DAY 57
Soothing Rhythms

PLACE A HAND OVER YOUR HEART. BEGIN GENTLY TAPPING WITH your hand. Then transition into making small circles as you rub or massage your sternum. Notice which movement is more comfortable or soothing. This is an easy way to identify a rhythm that soothes you during times of stress. You can then allow the rhythm to migrate all over your body.

DAY 58
Pat, Pat, Pat

STARTING AT THE TOP OF YOUR HEAD, BEGIN GENTLY PATTING YOUR hands over the surface of your body. As you make your way down to your feet, notice which parts of your body enjoy this sensation and which ones do not.

DAY 59
Making Sense

BRING TO MIND AN INSTANCE OR SITUATION WHEN SOMETHING JUST made sense to you. Essentially, it's when you agreed with or could logically understand an idea or thought that you or someone else suggested. Identify what "making sense" feels like to your body. Where does this live or settle? How do you know when something makes sense in your body? You may notice a relaxing or settling in your chest, abdomen, or shoulders.

....
....
....
....
....
....
....
....

DAY 60
How Are You *Moving?*

NOW THAT YOU HAVE FOCUSED MORE ON YOUR SENSES, THE LANguage of your body, take this time to check in with your awareness of your current movement. Again, notice how this has changed since you began. What senses are you most familiar with, and which ones need more attention?

....
....
....
....
....
....
....
....
....
....
....
....
....
....
....
....
....

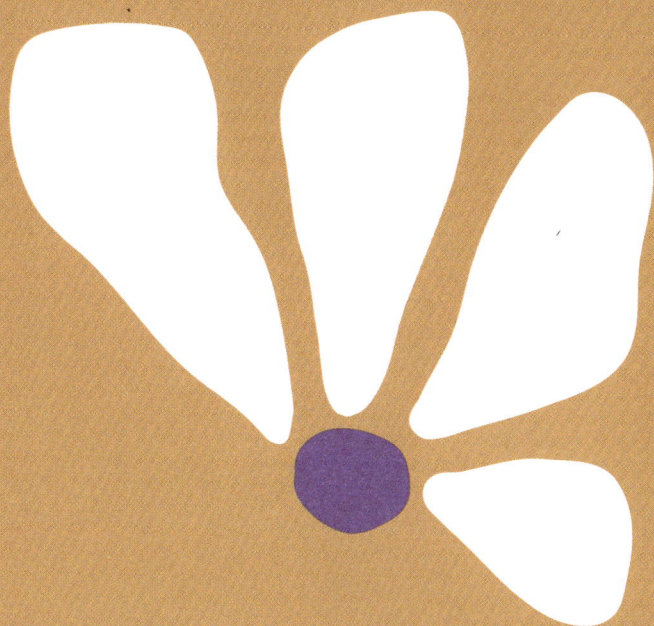

REGULATION

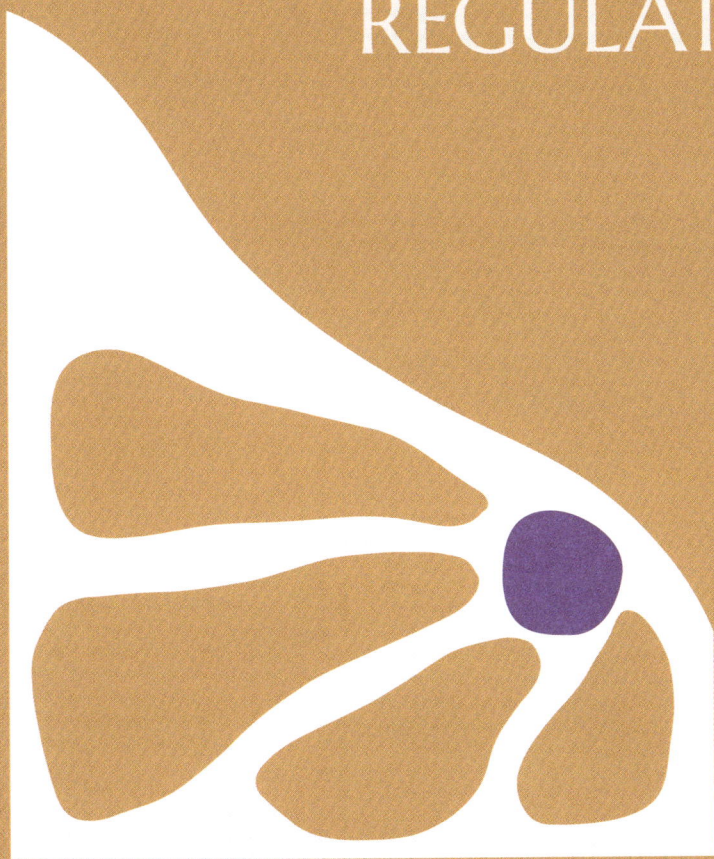

**Your state of mind
is a reflection of the
state of your body.**

DAY 61
Wiggle

BEGIN GENTLY WIGGLING YOUR TOES AND FINGERS. ALLOW THE movement to migrate through your body, up your arms, up your legs, until eventually your entire body is engaged in a wiggle.

DAY 62
Shake It Out

BEGINNING WITH THE WIGGLE FROM THE PREVIOUS DAY, SEE whether you can intensify the movement until it becomes a shake. Shake your hands, head, shoulders, hips, and everything in between. Shake off everything you've been carrying. Notice how you feel directly after the shake. Reflect on how your body feels compared with how it felt before you began this exercise.

....

....

....

....

....

....

....

....

....

....

DAY 63
Gentle Touch

GENTLY PRESS THE INDEX AND MIDDLE FINGERS OF EITHER HAND TO your lips. Place gentle pressure for ten to fifteen seconds, then release and repeat five times or more as needed.

Next, gently massage the outer cartilage of your ear.

Both these areas have nerve endings that connect to the vagus nerve, which signals the "rest and digest" reflex.

DAY 64
Legs Up

LIE DOWN ON A FIRM SURFACE WITH YOUR LEGS UP and resting on either the wall or a chair. Your legs should be well supported and your muscles should make little to no effort to hold them in place. Relax in this position for at least two or three minutes. Relax your arms on your abdomen or by your sides while you breathe gently into your belly. This position reduces cortisol levels, aids in digestion, and supports circulation.

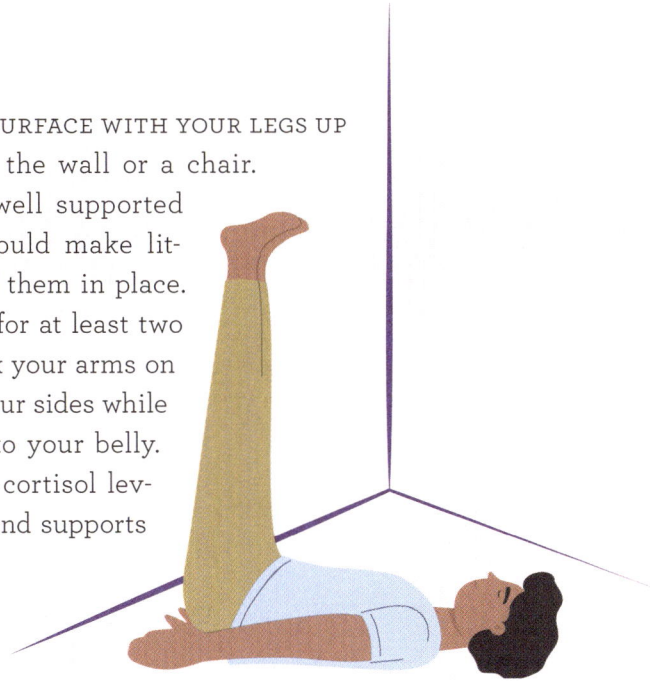

DAY 65
Create Sound

HUM OR SING A SONG. BOTH ARE WONDERFUL WAYS TO TONE THE vagus nerve, which signals the parasympathetic nervous system, which is responsible for reducing stress and enhancing calm.

DAY 66
Cradle Your Head

PLACE ONE HAND GENTLY ON YOUR FOREHEAD AND REST THE OTHER hand gently at the base of your skull. Apply gentle pressure with both hands. Take three cleansing breaths in through your nose and out through your mouth as you cradle your head and release tension.

DAY 67
Rock and Sway Away

EITHER STANDING OR SITTING, ALLOW YOUR BODY TO SLOWLY ROCK or sway. This can be done side to side or forward and back.

DAY 68
Drop It

LIFTING YOURSELF SLIGHTLY ONTO YOUR TOES, DROP YOUR HEELS TO the ground. Repeat five to ten times.

DAY 69
Tap It!

TAP YOUR FINGERTIPS TO THE THUMB ON THE SAME HAND. YOU CAN alternate hands or move both simultaneously. Play with different speeds and rhythms.

DAY 70
Four-Seven-Eight

THIS BREATHING TECHNIQUE ENGAGES THE PARASYMPATHETIC NERvous system to enhance calm and ease stress. Breathe in through your nose for a count of four. Hold your breath for a count of seven. Exhale out of your mouth for a count of eight.

Adjust the counts as needed to support your own breathing needs, making sure that the exhale is longer than the inhale and the hold.

DAY 71
Snake Breath

TAKE A CLEANSING BREATH IN THROUGH YOUR NOSE. AS YOU exhale, make a hissing sound like a snake, slowly letting the air out through your mouth.

DAY 72

Make Your Neck Disappear

BRING YOUR SHOULDERS UP TOWARD YOUR EARLOBES, INCREASING the tension as they rise. Hold for a count of three, then drop your shoulders as you exhale or sigh. Repeat three to five times.

DAY 73
Ball Toss

FIND A BALL OR SOMETHING ROUND, OPTIMALLY THE SIZE OF A TEN-nis ball or baseball. Gently toss the ball between your hands. Engage in this activity for three to five minutes or until you begin to feel a shift in your mood.

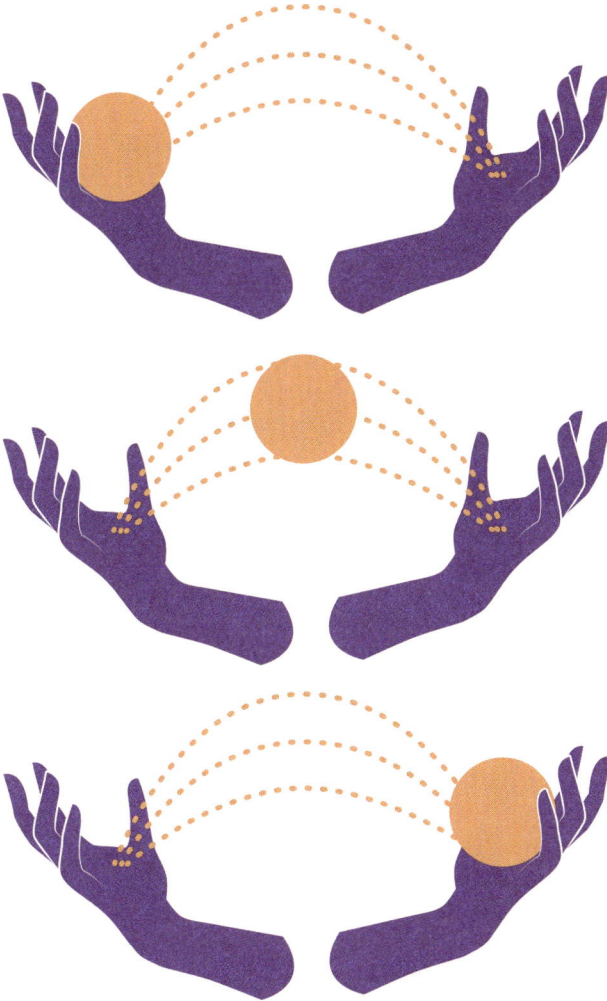

DAY 74
Interlace to Embrace

INTERLACE YOUR FINGERS. GENTLY PLACE YOUR HANDS ON THE crown of your head with your elbows gently pressing out to the side. Sit or stand as you breathe in through your nose and out through your mouth. With each exhale, allow the shoulders to draw down and away from your earlobes.

DAY 75
Energizing Breath

PLACE A HAND ON YOUR STERNUM. GENTLY APPLY PRESSURE AS YOU breathe into your hand. Release any tension in your torso as you exhale. This practice serves a dual purpose: It can up- or downregulate your nervous system depending on your needs in the moment. Repeat for two or three minutes or until you feel a shift in your body.

DAY 76
Progressive Muscle Relaxation

TAKE A MOMENT TO IDENTIFY A PART OF YOUR BODY THAT IS TENSE or tight. To a count of three, tighten that part intentionally, then release the tenseness. Repeat three times for each tense part you identify.

DAY 77
Sigh

TAKE A DEEP, CLEANSING BREATH IN THROUGH YOUR NOSE. AS YOU exhale out your mouth, add a sigh. Repeat this exercise three to five times. Notice any changes in your mood or the state of your body.

DAY 78
Toss a Pillow

STAND WITH YOUR FEET ABOUT HIP WIDTH APART AND WITH A SLIGHT bend in your knees. Reach a pillow above your head and then slam it onto the floor in front of you. Feel free to add a cleansing breath or sigh with each repetition. This is especially beneficial for releasing anger and intense feelings. Repeat five to ten times.

DAY 79
Drop Your Jaw

ALLOW YOUR JAW TO OPEN. YOU MAY FIND IT HELPFUL TO USE YOUR hands to massage the jaw muscles as you drop your jaw. Repeat three to five times. Notice any tension you may have been carrying in this part of your body.

DAY 80
X Marks the Spot

STANDING OR LYING DOWN, STRETCH YOUR BODY OUT INTO A LARGE X. Increase the stretch on your inhale and release it on the exhale. Allow your body to expand and contract naturally. Practice this exercise for three to five minutes.

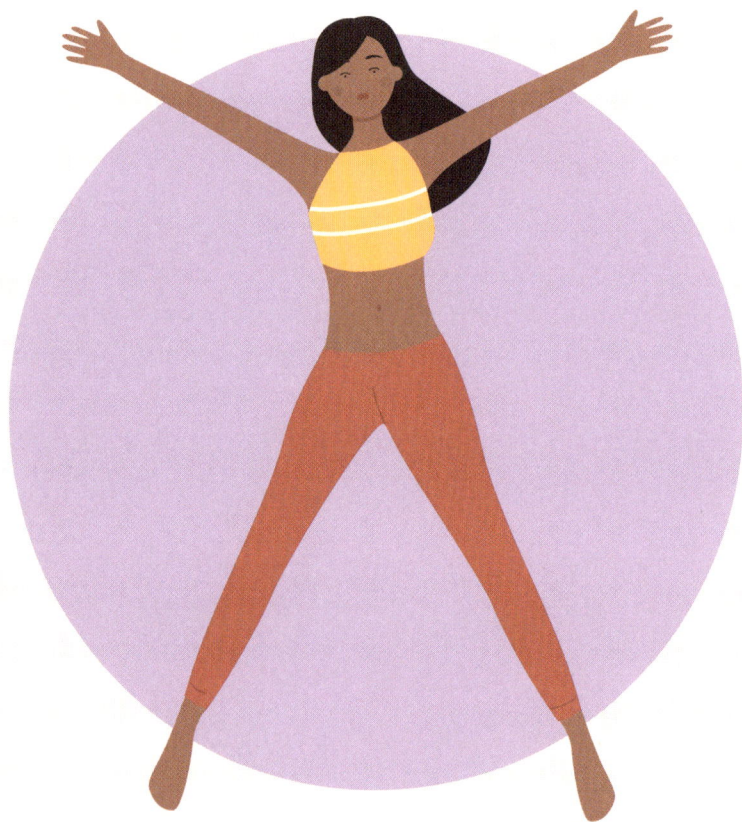

DAY 81
Happy Baby

LIE ON YOUR BACK AND BRING YOUR KNEES TO YOUR CHEST. REACH
up between your knees and grab your toes or ankles. Allow your body
to gently rock side to side.

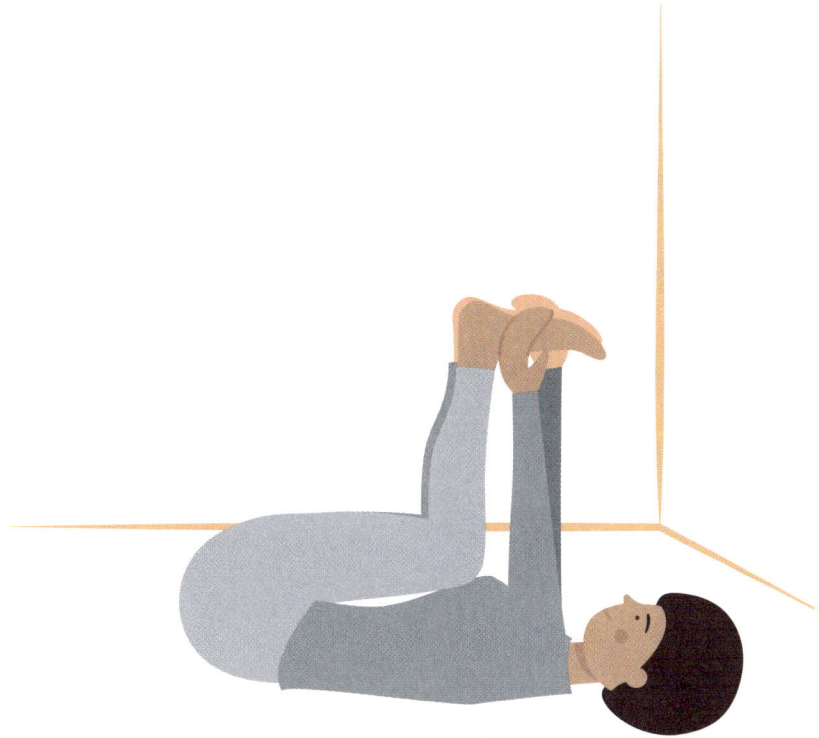

DAY 82
Child's Pose

KNEEL ON THE FLOOR ON ALL FOURS. SLOWLY BRING YOUR BOTTOM down onto your heels. Then move your chest toward the floor while allowing your knees to spread apart as you reach forward with your hands and place them on the floor in front of you. Let your forehead rest on the floor.

DAY 83
Hand Skating

BRING YOUR PALMS TOGETHER. SLIDE ONE HAND down and bring the fingertips toward your forearm while allowing the arm to extend to the side. Then slowly slide that hand back up to a prayer position and repeat on the other side.

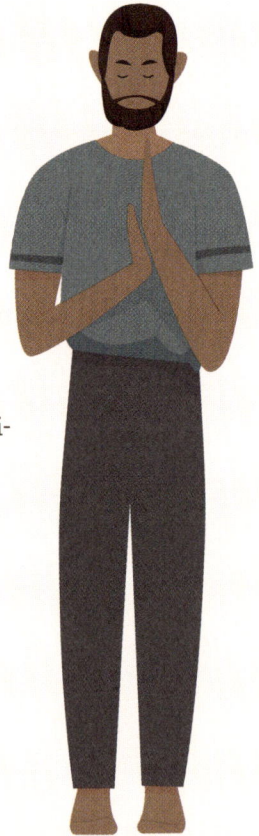

DAY 84
Move Your Hips

IT HAS BEEN SAID THAT HIPS HOLD EMOTIONS. TAKE TWO OR THREE minutes to move your hips. Here are some movements to try on:

Sway or rock
Thrust forward and back
Circle or Hula-Hoop
Make a figure eight
Wag your tail

DAY 85
Stretch Break

TAKE ONE MINUTE TO STRETCH YOUR BODY IN ANY WAY POSSIBLE. Notice what happens to your breathing pattern. How does stretching affect your thoughts or overall mood?

....
....
....
....
....
....
....
....

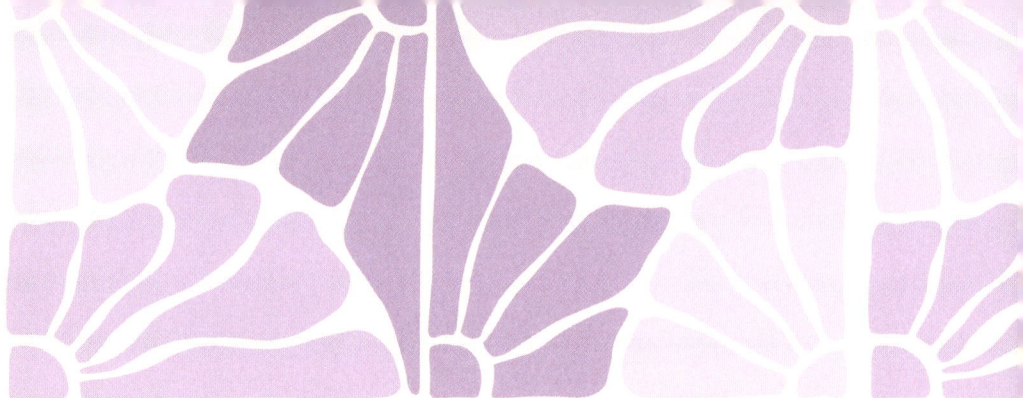

DAY 86
Brush It Off

BEGIN BRUSHING OFF YOUR SHOULDERS AS IF THERE WERE A BUG OR some dust there. Allow the brushing to migrate all over your body, alternating sides as needed.

DAY 87
Roll Your Shoulders

PLACE EACH HAND ON THE SHOULDER ON THE SAME SIDE. DRAW CIR-cles in the air with your elbows. Circle three times in each direction.

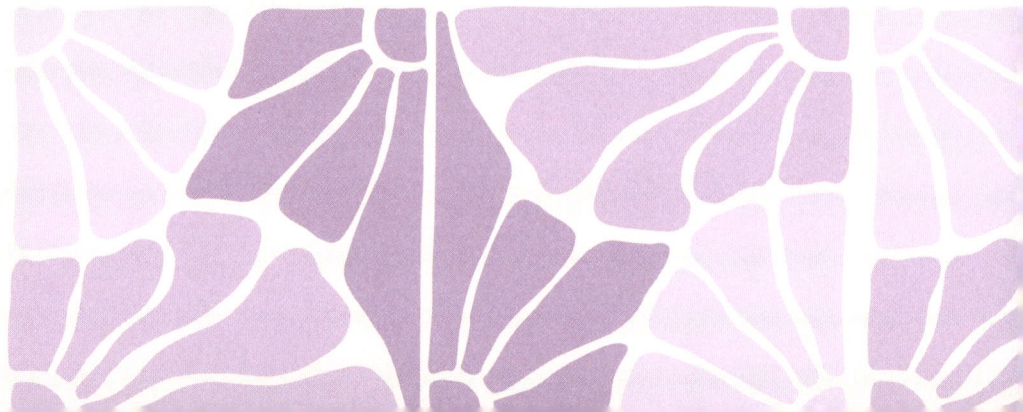

DAY 88
Root Yourself

PLACE YOUR FEET ON THE FLOOR AND STAND OR SIT IN AN UPRIGHT, lifted position. Imagine your feet as roots of a tree. Evenly distribute your weight from your toes to your heels.

DAY 89

Fingertip Press

PRESS YOUR FINGERTIPS INTO A COUNTERTOP, TABLE, OR DESK. GENtly apply pressure, feeling energy surge through your hands and up your arms. Hold this position for thirty seconds. Repeat three to five times or as needed.

DAY 90
How Are You *Moving?*

NOW IS THE TIME TO CHECK IN WITH HOW YOUR BODY IS MOVING. What new awareness do you have after engaging in practices of regulation? Make a list of the exercises that affected you the most. Save them on your computer or phone to use when you are feeling overwhelmed and stressed.

....

....

....

....

....

....

....

....

....

....

....

....

....

....

....

....

....

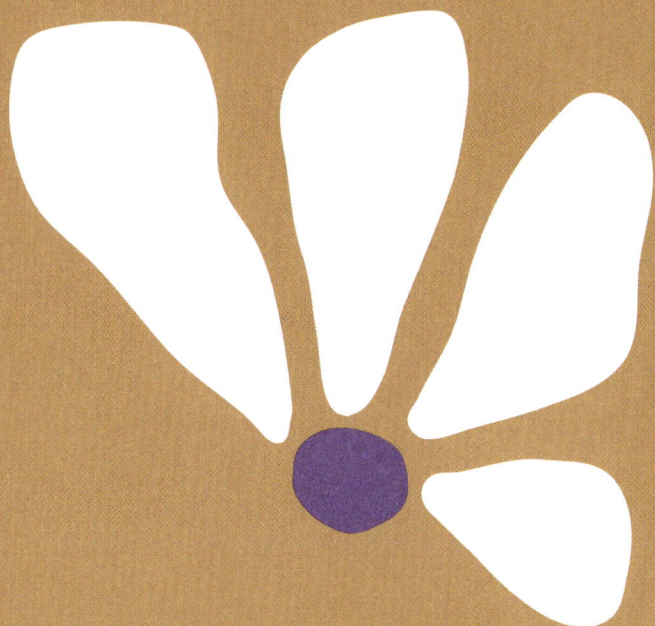

MOBILIZATION

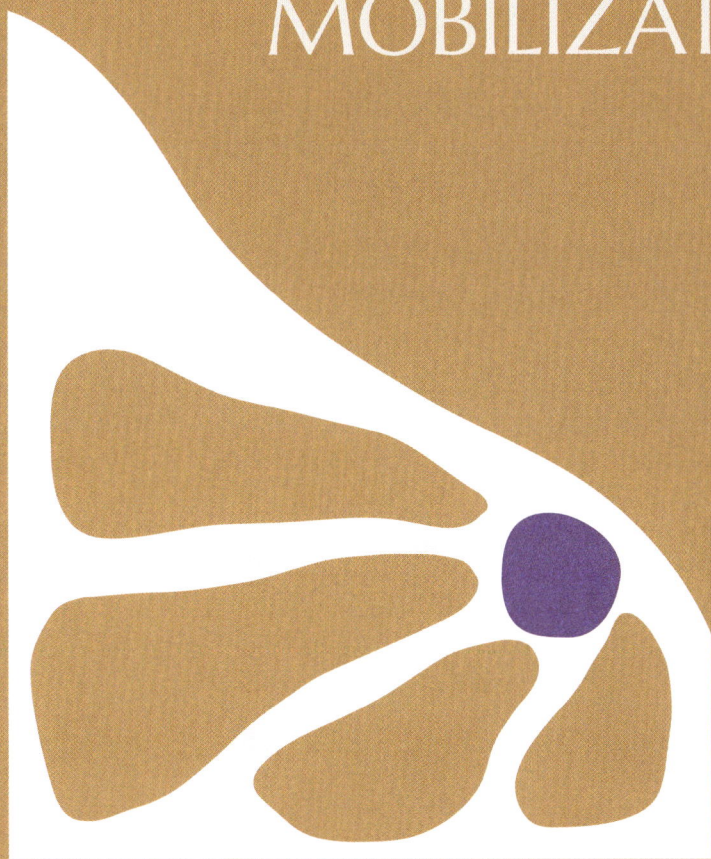

You are one movement away
from changing your mind.

DAY 91
Roll It Out

ROLL YOUR SHOULDERS BACKWARD THREE TIMES, THEN FORWARD three times. Repeat for two minutes or as needed throughout the day to relieve tension.

DAY 92
Head Turners

STAND WITH YOUR SHOULDERS AND HIPS POINTING FORWARD. RELAX your shoulders. Slowly turn your head toward your right shoulder, pass through center, and then turn toward your left shoulder. Allow your eyes to track straight ahead as you move your head back and forth. Repeat ten times.

DAY 93
Chin Up

LOOKING STRAIGHT AHEAD, DRAW YOUR CHIN UP TOWARD THE CEIL-ing while maintaining a long neck so as not to crunch the shoulders. Gently bring your chin down toward your chest. Repeat ten times.

DAY 94
Drawing Circles

IMAGINE YOUR NOSE IS A PENCIL, AND THE AIR IN FRONT OF YOU, A piece of paper. Draw a large circle in the air with your nose. Repeat three times in each direction (clockwise and counterclockwise).

DAY 95
Massage to Relax

WITH YOUR INDEX AND MIDDLE fingers on both hands, apply gentle pressure to your temples (the indentation on each side of your eyes). Now, make small circles as you massage this area. Next, move your fingers down your face to the large jaw muscles on each side. With your jaw relaxed, slowly massage the muscles with small circles.

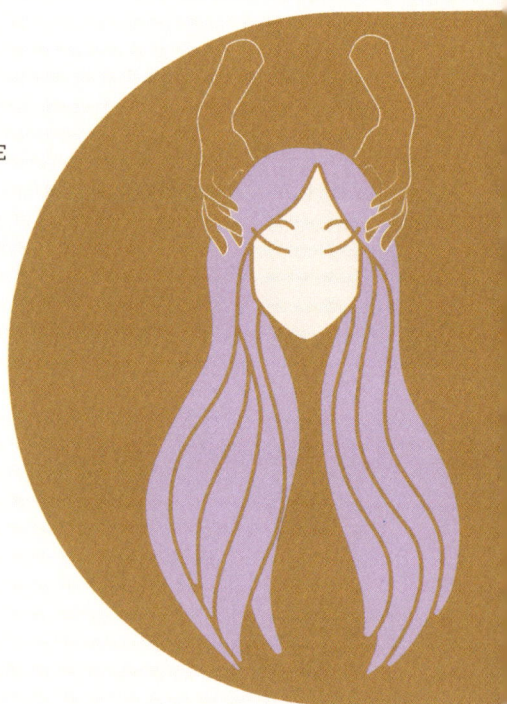

DAY 96
Get the Blood Flowing

USING THE FINGERTIPS ON BOTH HANDS, GENTLY TAP YOUR FORE-head. Allow your hands to tap down your cheeks toward your chin and back up again. Now move to the crown, sides, and back of your head. Notice how the surface of your head and face begin to feel more sensation and blood flow. How does this feel?

DAY 97
Wrist Circles

EITHER MAKE YOUR HANDS INTO FISTS OR WITH OPEN PALMS, CIRCLE your wrists. Try moving them in different directions at different speeds and intensities until you feel the joints relaxing and creating more mobility.

DAY 98
Arm Circles

MAKE LARGE CIRCLES WITH YOUR ARMS. START WITH EACH ARM down by your side, then slowly raise your arms out in front and up toward the ceiling, and open them out toward the sides and back down to your legs. Repeat three times in each direction.

DAY 99
Twist Your Waist

Stand with your feet hip width apart and your hands on your hips. Begin engaging your waist by pointing your chest to the left side of your body. Move back through center and point your chest toward the right side of your body. Bring your arms down and repeat this motion, allowing your arms to gently swing side to side as you twist at your waist. Play with the size and speed of the twist until you identify a rhythm that feels playful and fluid.

DAY 100
Wide-Leg Stance

Stand and widen your feet to just beyond hip width apart. Rock your hips side to side. You may place your hands on your hips if this feels more stable.

DAY 101
Hip Circles

Circle your hips to the right three times and then circle your hips to the left three times. Now see whether you can alternate with each circle. Wiggle or shake your tail (bottom) when you are done.

DAY 102
Rock and Roll

ROCK YOUR HIPS FRONT TO BACK, CURLING YOUR TAILBONE TOWARD your forehead and away. This exercise can be done seated or standing depending on your body's abilities in the present moment.

DAY 103
Twist It Out

BEGIN TWISTING YOUR HIPS AND LOWER BODY, WAKING UP YOUR legs and feet. Let the momentum of the movement direct your arms and upper body in any way that feels energizing and rejuvenating.

DAY 104
Marching

MARCH IN PLACE, GENTLY LIFTING YOUR KNEES. ALLOW THE MARCH-ing to move you through space as you begin marching forward, back-ward, and sideways.

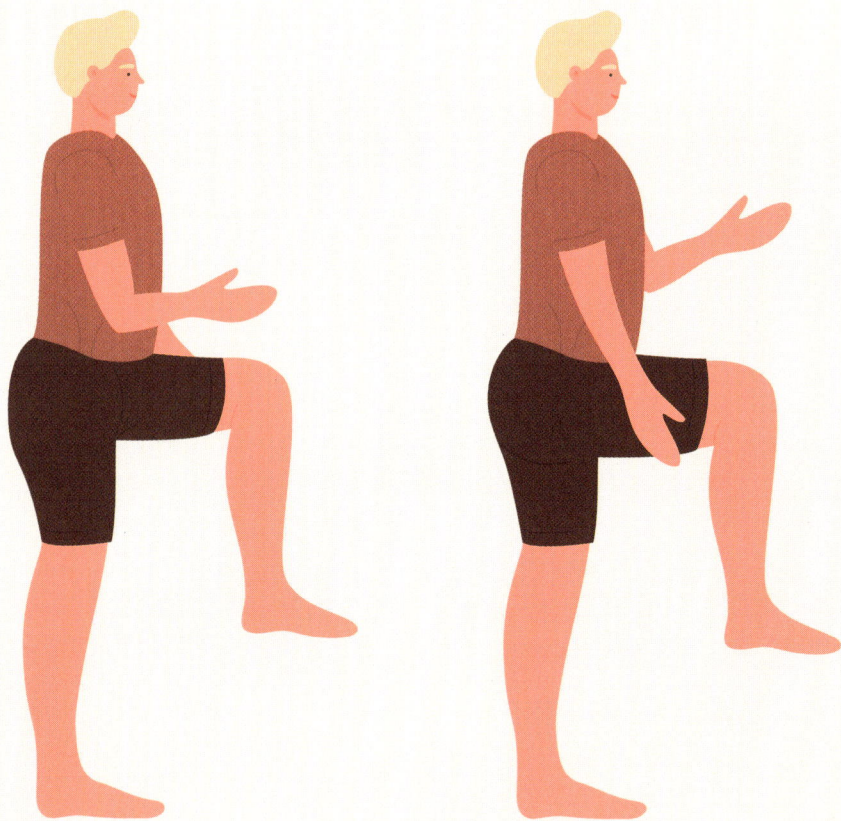

DAY 105
Jump Rope

PRETEND YOU ARE HOLDING A ROPE IN YOUR HANDS AND GENTLY jump rope, getting your feet just a few inches off the ground. Repeat ten to twenty times.

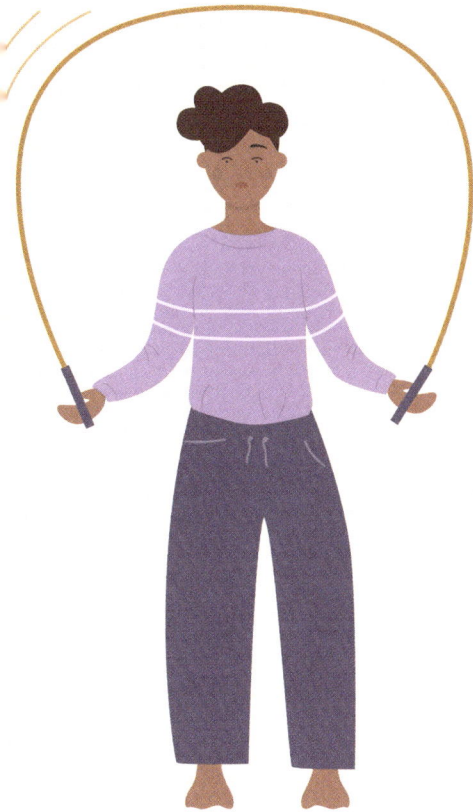

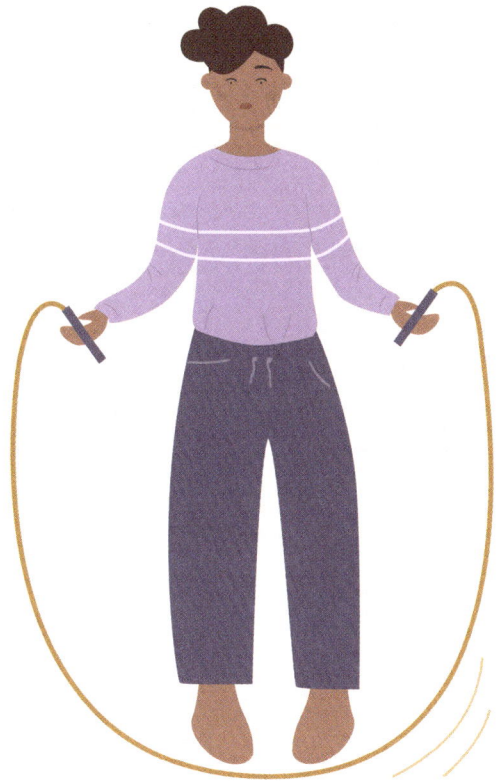

DAY 106
One Foot After Another

TAKE A WALK. BECOME AWARE OF HOW EACH FOOT MAKES CONTACT with the floor. With your heel making contact first, gently roll through your foot.

DAY 107

Point Your Toes

SIT DOWN AND STRETCH YOUR LEGS OUT IN FRONT OF YOU. POINT your toes across the room and flex your toes up toward the ceiling. You can alternate feet or move them simultaneously. Repeat this exercise fifteen to twenty times. Feel free to roll your ankles three to five times in each direction.

DAY 108
Knee Taps

IN A STANDING POSITION, BEGIN WITH YOUR LEGS IN A WIDE STANCE and your arms stretched out to the sides at about shoulder height. Hinging at the waist with a slight twist to the right, tap your left hand to your right knee. Repeat on the other side, alternating sides for one minute.

For those who prefer to stay seated, in a seated position, alternate tapping each knee with the opposite hand. Increase the range of motion by tapping lower on your leg or, hinging forward at the waist, tapping your toes. Repeat for one minute.

DAY 109
Reach

REACH YOUR ARMS INTO THE SPACE ABOVE YOUR HEAD. INHALE AS you reach up and exhale as you begin to reach down. Reach toward the space below your knees. Repeat this sequence three times.

DAY 110
Spine Twist

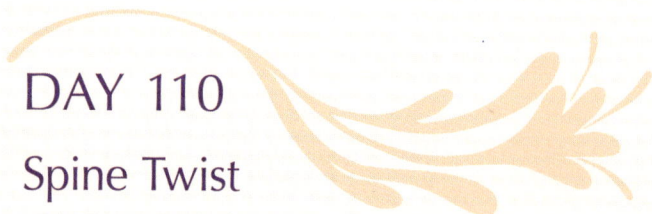

STANDING OR SITTING, DROP YOUR ARMS TO YOUR SIDES. BRING BOTH hands over to your left side, gently twisting at the waist as you look over your left shoulder. Repeat on the right side. Repeat this series three times.

DAY 111
Take Action

STANDING WITH YOUR FEET HIP WIDTH APART, MOVE FORWARD through the space in front of you. After a few steps, allow yourself to walk backward, exploring the space behind you.

DAY 112
Full-Body Breath

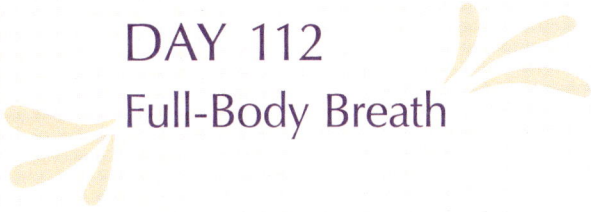

STAND WITH YOUR FEET WIDER THAN HIP WIDTH APART AND WITH A slight bend in your knees. Relax your arms at your sides. As you inhale, slowly bring your arms out to the sides and up over your head. As you exhale, bring your arms back down to your sides. Repeat three times, deepening your breath and stretch each time.

DAY 113
Your Choice

TAKE TIME TODAY TO ENGAGE IN A PHYSICAL ACTIVITY OF YOUR choice. This does not have to be exercise but could be anything that uses your body to take action, such as cooking, sewing, journaling, or walking.

....

....

....

....

....

....

....

....

....

DAY 114
Go with the Flow!

CHOOSE FIVE OF YOUR FAVORITE MOVEMENTS FROM THIS SECTION and create your own mobility flow. Incorporate them into your everyday routine.

1. ....
2. ....
3. ....
4. ....
5. ....

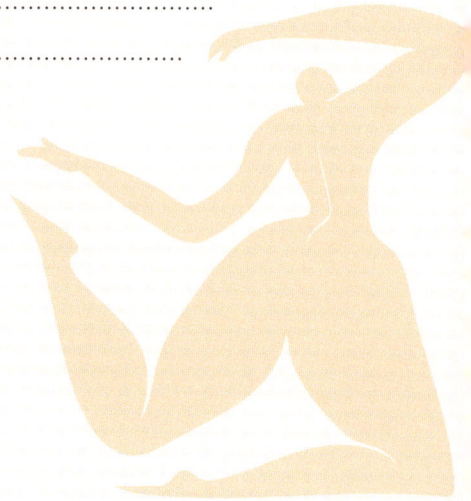

DAY 115
Your Stuck Parts

IDENTIFY A PLACE IN YOUR BODY THAT FEELS STUCK OR IMMOBILE. Begin massaging or touching that part until you are able to move it on its own. Allow the movement to migrate around the rest of your body.

DAY 116
Getting Unstuck

MAKE A LIST OF PLACES OR SITUATIONS WHERE YOU FEEL IMMOBILE
or stuck. This may be a job, a relationship, or a difficult problem. Consider how mobilizing your body will aid in mobilizing your thoughts
and cognitive processes. Make a list of movement interventions you
can try next time you feel emotionally stuck.

....

....

....

....

....

....

....

....

....

....

....

....

....

....

....

....

....

DAY 117
Spread Out

STAND IN A DOORWAY. REACH YOUR HANDS TOWARD THE TOP TWO corners and place your feet in the bottom two corners. Breathe into this position, allowing your body to take up space.

DAY 118
Be Vocal

MAKE A SOUND WITH YOUR VOICE. THIS CAN BE SPEAKING OUT LOUD, singing, humming, or whistling. Practice moving your vocal cords to mobilize your voice.

DAY 119
Stillness

TAKE THIRTY SECONDS, IF POSSIBLE, TO BE STILL. PAY ATTENTION TO the parts of you that are still moving. For example, your heart beating, diaphragm breathing, eyes moving. Write down all the ways your body moves even when it is static or practicing stillness.

What was hard about being still?

....

....

....

....

....

....

....

....

....

....

....

....

....

....

....

....

....

....

DAY 120
How Are You *Moving*?

TAKE TIME TO JOURNAL ABOUT HOW YOU ARE MOVING DIFFERENTLY since expanding your awareness around your mobility. Reflect on the following:

My "stuckness" shows up in my body through . . .

When I feel stuck emotionally, I can move physically by . . .

....
....
....
....
....
....
....
....
....
....
....
....
....
....
....
....

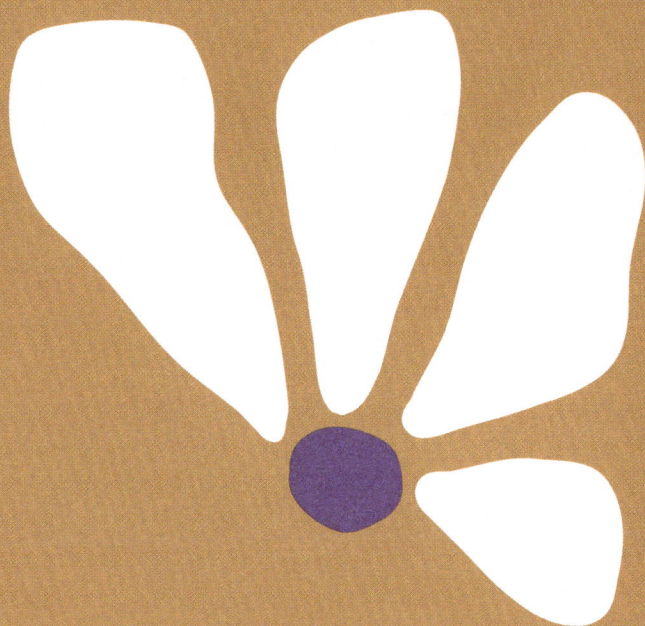

STABILIZATION AND BALANCE

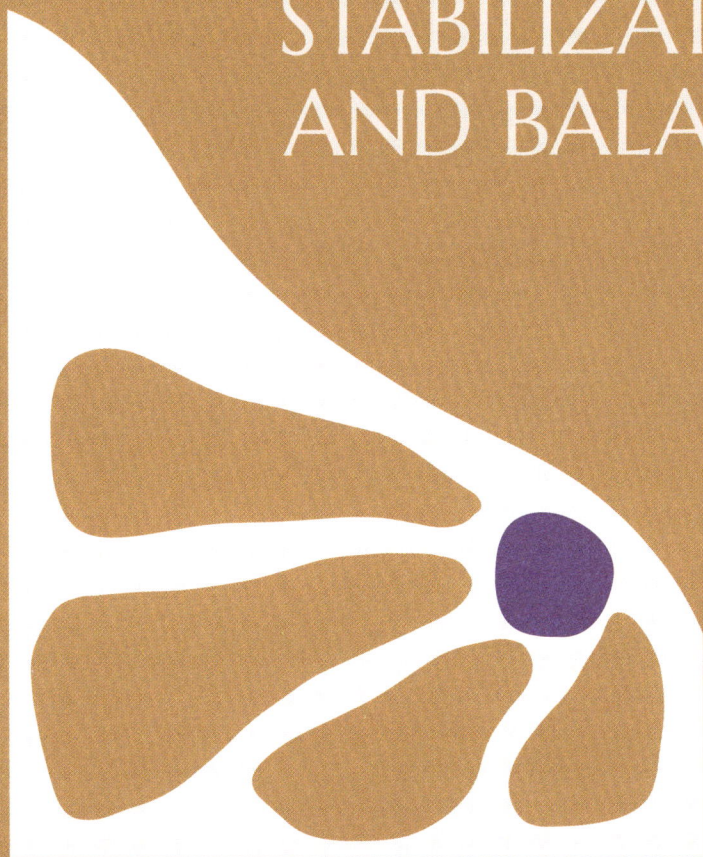

An anxious mind craves certainty, which comes from a sense of stability and security in the body.

DAY 121
Journaling Exercise

REFLECT FOR AT LEAST THREE MINUTES ON THE FOLLOWING QUES-
tions, then write down whatever comes to mind.

Where in my life do I feel established or stable?
Who in my life provides support and stability?
What challenges my sense of balance and control?

....

....

....

....

....

Next, reflect on how your movement and body respond to the
answers to the previous questions.

What are the movement characteristics (shape, time, space) present in these situations or with certain people?

....

....

....

....

....

DAY 122
Control

THINK ABOUT YOUR ASSOCIATION WITH THE WORD *CONTROL*. NOTICE any visceral, or felt, sensations in your body. Write down anything that comes to mind and body about *control*.

....

....

....

....

....

....

....

....

DAY 123
Embodying Control

REVIEW THE PREVIOUS DAY'S REFLECTION. THEN, FIND A WAY TO embody or bring a physical representation of what you define as *control* into your movement.

How does this feel?

....
....

What do I notice?

....
....

Do I feel grounded?

....
....

How does a false sense of control in the body affect my mind?

....
....

DAY 124
Losing Control

TAKE A MOMENT TO REFLECT ON WHAT *OUT OF CONTROL* MEANS TO you. Write down all the ways emotionally, cognitively, and physically you might perceive yourself or someone else being out of control. Notice the movement characteristics present in this movement or body posture. Journal about your thoughts.

....
....
....
....
....
....
....
....
....
....
....
....
....
....
....
....
....
....
....
....
....

DAY 125
Feeling Support

LIE DOWN ON A FIRM SURFACE, IDEALLY A HARDWOOD OR CARPETED floor. Feel free to use a light blanket, towel, or yoga mat to ease any discomfort. Allow your legs to stretch out and arms to rest naturally at your sides. Give yourself permission to close your eyes as you allow the floor to support you. With each exhale, let the pressure or tension in your body melt into the floor.

DAY 126

Calming Breaths

RESTING COMFORTABLY ON THE FLOOR, BRING YOUR KNEES TOWARD your chest and gently hold your knees with your hands. Slowly breathe into your belly and allow your body to gently rock side to side. Repeat at least five times before coming back to the knee-holding position. Repeat the entire exercise as needed to create a sense of calm in your body and mind.

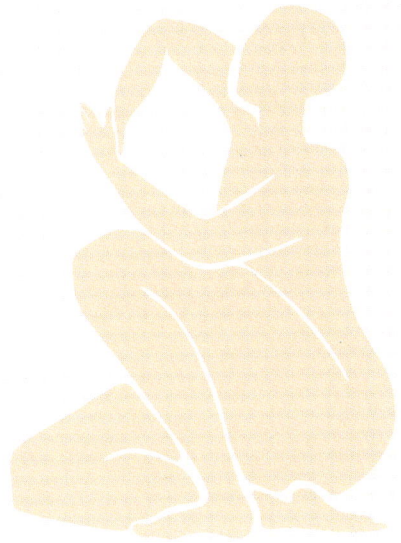

DAY 127
Moving X

BEGIN BY LYING ON THE FLOOR WITH YOUR ARMS AND LEGS MAKING a giant X. Slowly glide your right knee and elbow toward each other, maintaining contact with the floor as best you can. Allow this movement to roll you over to your right side. Tuck your head and tail as you bring your body into a fetal position.

Slowly return to the giant X by swooping your left arm above your head and your left leg out and down. Pause, take a breath in this giant X, and repeat on the left side.

Repeat this exercise until you feel more fluid in the transition from side to side.

DAY 128
Roll Around

LIE ON THE FLOOR. IMAGINE THE FLOOR IS COVERED IN WET PAINT and your body is the canvas. Allow your body to slowly roll around in any way or direction it feels compelled. Try covering the canvas with as much paint as possible as you maneuver on the floor, covering all the crevices, curves, and lines of your body.

DAY 129
Rest and Digest

LIE DOWN ON YOUR STOMACH. PLACE YOUR FOREHEAD ON THE BACK of your hands as your elbows rest out to the sides. Breathe deeply into your belly, feeling your lower back expand with air. Think about drawing your shoulder blades down your back and away from your ears as you exhale.

DAY 130
Roll the Marble

LYING ON YOUR STOMACH, BEND YOUR ELBOWS AND PLACE YOUR hands directly under your shoulders. Press your hands and forearms into the floor and gently lift your upper body, beginning with the crown of your head. Think about slowly rolling a marble down your spine no farther than your mid-back. Pause here and take two cleansing breaths in through the nose, out through the mouth. Gently return to the starting position.

Repeat this exercise two more times. On the third time, gently move your head right to left, then left to right.

DAY 131
Cat Stretch

COME ONTO YOUR HANDS AND KNEES. PLACE YOUR KNEES HIP WIDTH apart and your hands directly under your shoulders. Gently push your hands into the floor and slowly curl or round your spine while tucking your chin. Slowly return to your original position.

DAY 132
Cow

COMING ONTO YOUR HANDS AND KNEES AGAIN, ALLOW YOUR SPINE to arch in a downward curve, with your belly pushing toward the floor. Imagine the crown of your head reaching for your tailbone. Return to the original position. You can revisit cat stretch and move between the two. This gentle exercise, also known as the cat-cow sequence in yoga practice, supports fluidity of the spine as well as a head–tail connection that supports stability, mobility, and self-awareness.

DAY 133
Be a Tree

STAND WITH YOUR FEET HIP WIDTH APART, knees slightly bent, and shoulders directly over your hips. Imagine someone gently pulling a string that comes out the top of your head. Feel your spine lengthen and your shoulders press down away from your ears as your arms rest comfortably at your sides. Imagine your legs are the trunk of a tree, and with each exhale, allow the roots of the tree to extend farther and farther into the ground. Slowly breathe into your belly.

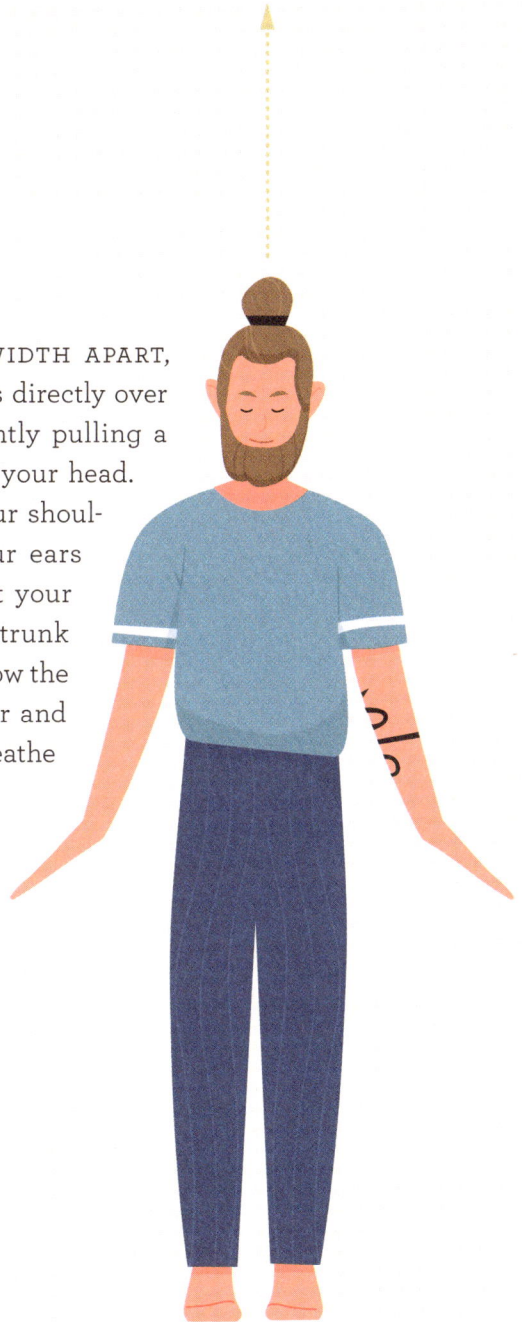

DAY 134
Find Your Stability

FIND WAYS TO STABILIZE YOURSELF THROUGHOUT THE DAY. FOR example, while brushing your teeth, cooking your breakfast, or making your morning coffee, plant your feet on the floor and gently press your hands onto the countertop or gently hold onto a counter for support. Be sure you do not grip or brace but rather gently hold or press. Look for ways to reinforce this throughout your day.

DAY 135
On All Fours

EXPLORE WHAT IT FEELS LIKE TO CRAWL AROUND. BE SURE TO TAKE care of your knees and wrists, because this exercise can put strain on them. You may want to wear some padding on your knees and shake out or roll your wrists as needed.

When was the last time I crawled?

....

....

How does this feel?

....

....

What does this remind me of?

....

....

DAY 136
Pick Yourself Up

BEGIN BY LYING DOWN ON THE FLOOR IN ANY POSITION THAT FEELS comfortable to you. Using some of the previous explorations, make your way to standing. The goal isn't to stand immediately but rather to explore the ways you can support yourself as you come to standing. This practice should be done slowly and intentionally. Set a timer, if needed, for three minutes and use all that time to come to an upright position.

What was difficult about this exercise?

....

....

What was easy about it?

....

....

How did it feel to find support as I picked myself up off the floor?

....

....

DAY 137
Wall Work

STAND FACING A WALL OR CLOSED DOOR (ENSURE THE DOOR WILL not open, because you will be leaning against it). Place your hands on the wall in front of you, with your arms outstretched, soft elbows, and feet flat on the floor hip width apart. Slowly begin to lean into the wall, maintaining contact with your hands. Allow yourself to feel the pressure and stability as the wall supports your body weight. Gently press away, maintaining connection with the wall as you return to your original position. Repeat three times.

DAY 138
Wall Lean

WITH YOUR FEET ABOUT TWO FEET OUT FROM THE WALL, LEAN YOUR back against the wall (or door). Feel the pressure along your back as the wall supports your body. Reflect on how it feels to be supported.

DAY 139
Contact Improv

LEAN AGAINST A WALL IN WHATEVER WAY FEELS MOST STABLE FOR you. Imagine the wall being covered with wet paint. Slowly begin covering your body with the paint as you maneuver around the wall, maintaining a connection with the wall and at least one part of your body at all times.

DAY 140
Walk Away

START BY LEANING INTO OR AGAINST THE WALL. SLOWLY WALK AWAY as you gradually disengage from the wall. Become aware of what your body needs to feel grounded, balanced, and stable as you leave the support of the wall and learn to support yourself.

DAY 141

Finding Your Balance

BEGIN IN A STANDING POSITION WITH YOUR FEET WELL GROUNDED on the floor. Allow your body to slowly sway side to side. As your center of gravity shifts, allow your body to fall off center and return. Less is more. The goal isn't to fall off-balance but to gain a sense of balance and stability.

DAY 142

Walking in Space

BEGIN WALKING THROUGH THE SPACE AROUND YOU. WALK SLOWLY to practice maintaining your balance. Change the speed as needed to feel stable and to challenge your balance when you feel ready.

DAY 143
Slow Walking

BUILDING ON THE PREVIOUS EXERCISE, BEGIN SLOWLY WALKING. TRY with each step to lift your knee slightly as you balance on the other leg before putting that foot down and moving on to the next step.

DAY 144
Heel Lifts

STAND IN A FIRM AND GROUNDED POSITION WITH YOUR FEET HIP width apart. Gently rise onto the balls of your feet, lifting your heels off the floor. Repeat this exercise ten times.

DAY 145
Heel Lifts Revisited

BEGIN WITH THE PREVIOUS EXERCISE. ON THE FIFTH REPETITION, stay lifted on your toes and hold this position for ten to twenty seconds. Become aware of any wobbling in your ankles. If you find it difficult to maintain stability in your ankles, release the hold and continue with the previous exercise.

DAY 146
On Your Toes?

COME ONTO THE BALLS OF YOUR FEET. CLOSE YOUR EYES AND MAIN-
tain this hold for thirty to sixty seconds. If this is easy, challenge yourself by extending the recommended time.

How does this change my feeling of stability?

....
....
....
....
....
....
....
....
....
....
....
....
....
....
....
....
....
....

DAY 147
On One Leg

STAND NEXT TO OR IN FRONT OF A TABLE OR COUNTER. BEGINNING in your grounded stance, with your feet hip width apart, slowly lift one knee as you balance on the other leg. The height of your knee is not nearly as important as maintaining your center and stability. Try to maintain this position, gently holding onto the table or counter if needed, for twenty seconds. Repeat three times on each leg.

DAY 148
On One Leg Revisited

REPEAT THE PREVIOUS DAY'S EXERCISE. IF IT IS STILL CHALLENGING, increase the duration to thirty seconds. If you find this exercise easy, try the same thing but with your eyes closed.

DAY 149
One Step at a Time

IN THIS FAST-PACED WORLD, SOMETIMES WE NEED A GOOD REMINDER to slow down and literally take things one step at a time. Take three to five minutes to simply walk with one foot in front of the other, strategically and methodically. Resist the urge to speed up, and keep a steady pace while you maintain balance and posture. This can be executed inside or outside. Be sure that your immediate space is free from obstructions or obstacles.

DAY 150
How Are You *Moving?*

REFLECT ON THE LAST THIRTY DAYS. JOURNAL ON YOUR EXPERI-
ences around stability and balance. What have you come to real-
ize about the connection between emotional stability and physical
balance?

....

....

....

....

....

....

....

....

....

....

....

....

....

....

....

....

....

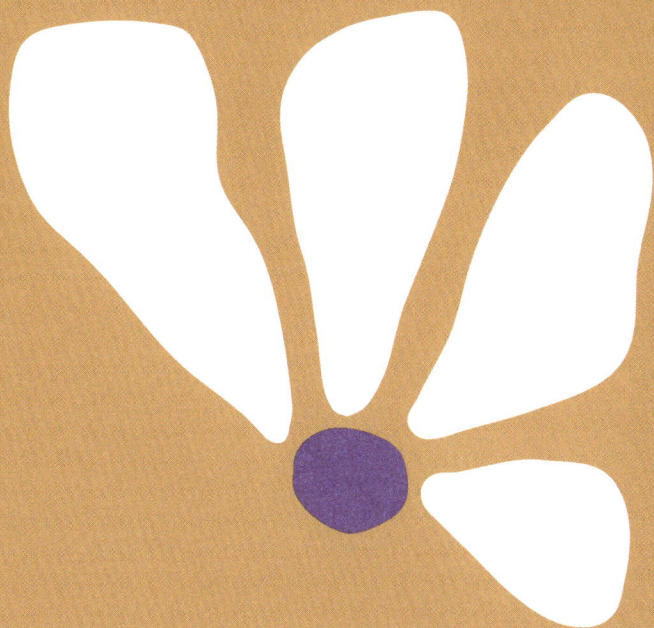

CONNECTION

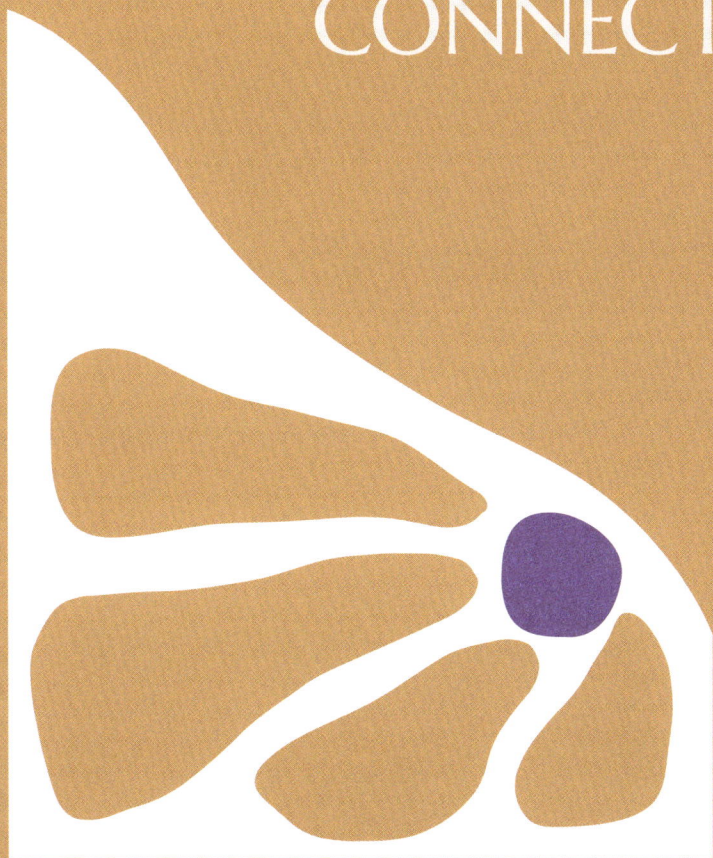

When the mind craves
attention, the body
requires connection.

DAY 151
Rest

THIS IS YOUR PERMISSION TO TAKE A BREAK FROM INTENTIONALLY connecting to your body. Here's an important note: Your mind doesn't need to be listening to hear your body speak. Your body is always talking. This is a day to rest from the intentional healing and an opportunity to just be.

DAY 152
Disconnect

SAY THIS WORD OUT LOUD AND NOTICE WHERE IT LANDS IN YOUR body: *Disconnect*. Ironically, you are making space and creating awareness around your connection to how it feels to be disconnected, unattached, maybe even free in some ways.

DAY 153
Take a Walk Without Distractions

TAKE A WALK FOR AT LEAST FIFTEEN MINUTES, MORE IF YOU ARE able, without any technology. The goal is to disconnect from any distractions, such as phones, music, and podcasts, and to connect to the sights and sounds in your surroundings.

DAY 154
Journaling

CONSIDER AND RESPOND TO THE FOLLOWING PROMPTS:

I feel most connected to myself when . . .

....
....
....

To others when . . .

....
....
....

To the environment when . . .

....
....
....

What makes it difficult to be or feel connected?

....
....
....

DAY 155
Likes and Dislikes

ASK YOURSELF THE FOLLOWING QUESTIONS:

What do I like? How do I feel when I like something?

....

....

....

What don't I like? How do I know I do not like something?

....

....

....

DAY 156
Embody Connection

TAKE FIVE MINUTES TO JOURNAL ON WHAT CONNECTION MEANS TO you.

On the basis of your writing, find a way to express through movement, posture, or gesture what connection looks or feels like.

....

....

....

....

....

DAY 157

Safe Connection

REFLECT ON WHAT YOUR BODY NEEDS TO FEEL SAFE TO CONNECT with others.

....

....

....

....

....

DAY 158
Eye Contact

EYE CONTACT IS AN IMPORTANT ASPECT OF CONNECTION. THE NEXT time you are speaking with someone face-to-face, practice making eye contact. Take the opportunity to make intentional eye contact with someone today. It may be a coworker, a barista, or even a stranger passing by. Notice how long you can maintain eye contact before either person looks away or feels the need to divert from it. Identify the sweet spot in terms of appropriate length of time for you to make a connection with the person and not just the words they are saying. What happens in your body when the other person meets your gaze? Are you able to maintain eye contact?

....

....

....

....

....

....

....

....

....

....

DAY 159
Take a Screen Break

SET A TIMER FOR FIVE MINUTES. DISCONNECT FROM ANY SCREENS OR technology during this time. Reflect on how and what you feel in the absence of screens.

....
....
....
....
....
....
....
....
....
....
....
....
....
....
....
....
....
....

DAY 160
Take Yourself on a Date

MAKE TIME FOR YOURSELF. WHETHER IT'S A MEAL, A MOVIE, OR SIM-
ply a walk, prioritize the connection to yourself.

What emerges as I carve out space for "me" time?

....

....

....

How does it feel to be with myself?

....

....

....

*How do I feel about the current connection I have with
myself?*

....

....

....

DAY 161
Reconnect with a Friend

FRIENDSHIP IS NECESSARY AT ALL AGES, AND OFTEN IT'S HARDER TO make new friends as we get older. Consider connecting with an old friend or someone with whom you haven't spoken in a long time. (Not someone you had a falling out or conflict with.) Identify the best way for you to reach out, whether that is by phone, email, or text. Notice how you feel as you think about reconnecting with this person. If this feeling is comforting, exciting, or joyful, take the steps to reach out.

DAY 162
Feed Someone

CONNECT WITH SOMEONE THROUGH A MEAL. INVITE SOMEONE OVER to your home or out for a meal or coffee. This is an opportunity to connect over a shared meal.

DAY 163
Dance with Someone

CONNECT WITH SOMEONE THROUGH A SHARED RHYTHM. THIS CAN be a loved one, a friend, or even a stranger in a safe place. Some ideas are to have an impromptu dance party in your kitchen, a night out at a club, or a formal ballroom dancing class.

What feelings come up for me around dancing?

....

....

....

What about dancing in front of or with others?

....

....

....

DAY 164
Be Someone's Mirror

MIRRORING SOMEONE IS A WAY TO CREATE EMPATHY AND UNDER-standing on a body level. You might mirror someone's posture in passing, while sharing a meal, or in a conversation or meeting. Mirroring involves reflecting what you are seeing, not mocking or mimicking the person. Invite someone into this experience with you. Have a conversation about what it was like for both of you.

DAY 165
What Do You Need?

IDENTIFY FIVE NEEDS YOU HAVE RIGHT NOW. THESE CAN BE PHYSI-cal or emotional. Next, list one or two ways you can meet those needs. Last, allow yourself to meet any needs that can be addressed in the moment.

1. ....

2. ....

3. ....

4. ....

5. ....

DAY 166
Reach Out

INVITE YOURSELF TO CONTACT OR SEND A MESSAGE TO SOMEONE YOU have been following on social media. Identify someone with whom you have shared ideas or content. Keep in mind that larger accounts or influencers may not reciprocate. This is an opportunity to deepen a connection off of social media.

DAY 167
Self-Awareness

WHILE SITTING OR STANDING, BRING YOUR CHIN TO YOUR CHEST and slowly roll down your spine, guiding the crown of your head toward your lap or the floor. When you find a stopping point, slowly roll back up, identifying each vertebra, zipping your spine up, and coming back to a neutral position.

DAY 168
Priming Connection to Others

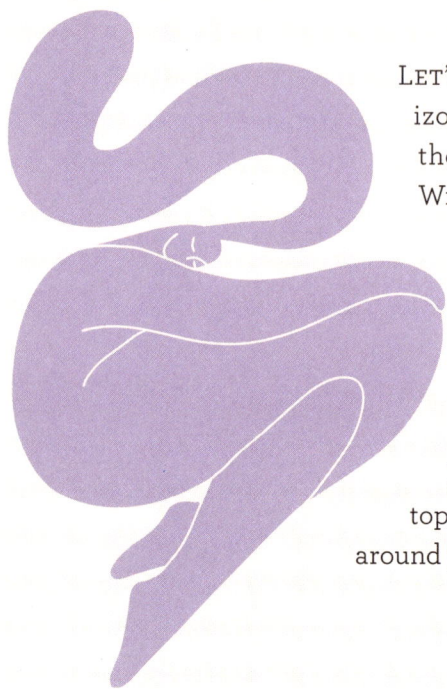

LET'S REVISIT CONNECTING TO THE HOR-izontal plane. This movement primes the body for connecting to others. Wrap your arms around your torso, giving yourself a big embrace. Next, stretch your arms out to the side. Allow your body to move in this dimension, also known as the table plane. Imagine yourself standing in the middle of a table. Move your arms across the table-top, twisting and wrapping your arms around your body.

DAY 169
Connect to Your Environment

MOVE THROUGH YOUR ENVIRONMENT IN A FORWARD AND BACK motion. Some examples can be walking forward and backward, rocking back and forth, or standing in a warrior pose. Moving in this plane, also called the sagittal or wheel plane, primes the body and mind for connection to the world around you.

DAY 170
Cross Your Midline

CROSSING THE MIDLINE OF YOUR BODY ENCOURAGES THE LEFT AND right hemispheres of your brain to communicate. Let's create connection across the corpus callosum (the band of fibers that unites the two cerebral hemispheres) in the following ways:

1. Interlace your fingers. Notice which thumb is on top. Place the other thumb on top and reposition your other fingers accordingly. Move between the two positions three to five times.

2. Cross your arms over your chest. Notice which arm is on top. Allow the other arm to come to the top. Move between the two positions three to five times.

3. Cross your legs at the knees or ankles. Practice crossing your legs both ways three to five times.

How does it feel when I cross my nondominant hand or leg?

....

....

....

....

....

....

....

....

....

DAY 171
Connect to Time

IDENTIFY AN ENVIRONMENT THAT FEELS SECURE, COMFORTABLE, and familiar in which to move about. This exercise can be done indoors or outside. Begin walking at a brisk pace. After thirty seconds, slow your pace. Play between the two speeds and explore what different timing feels like in your body.

Which is my natural time? Which feels most familiar?

....

....

....

Which pace do I need more of?

....

....

....

DAY 172
Connect to Space

BEGIN MOVING THROUGH YOUR ENVIRONMENT, MAKING SURE NOT to bump into or touch anything. Notice how it feels to limit your space. Next, clear your space or relocate to an area that will allow you to move freely without the fear of bumping into anything. Now take up more space, reaching and extending your body.

Which feels more familiar?

....
....
....

Which feels uncomfortable?

....
....
....

Which do I engage in most in my life?

....
....
....

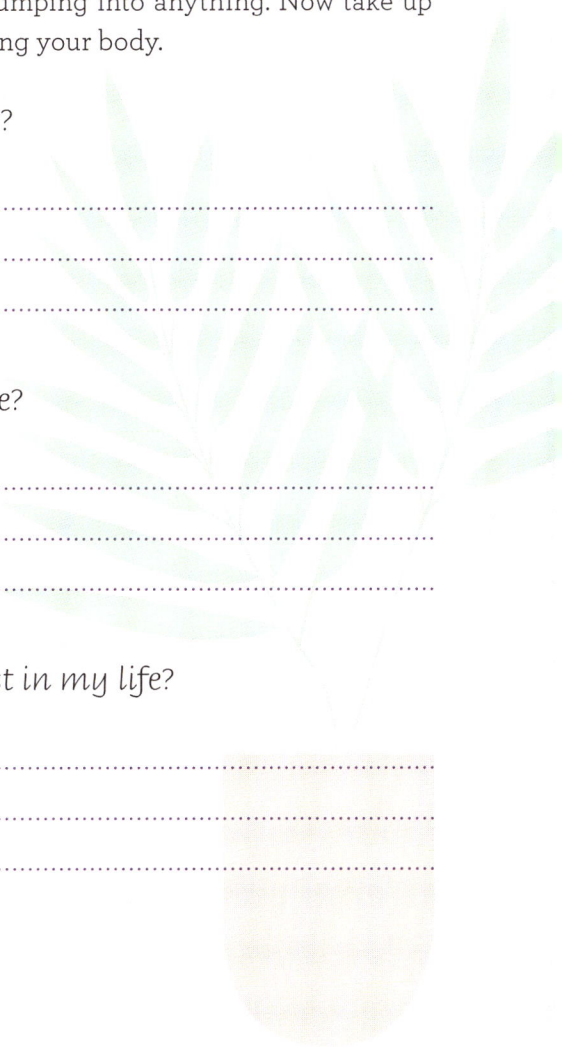

DAY 173
Connect with Nature

FIND WAYS TO CONNECT WITH NATURE. FOLLOWING ARE SOME examples:

> *Sway with the breeze.*
> *Shake with the leaves of the trees.*
> *Breathe in the fresh air.*
> *Watch the sunrise or sunset.*

You don't always need a person to coregulate. You can use Mother Nature.

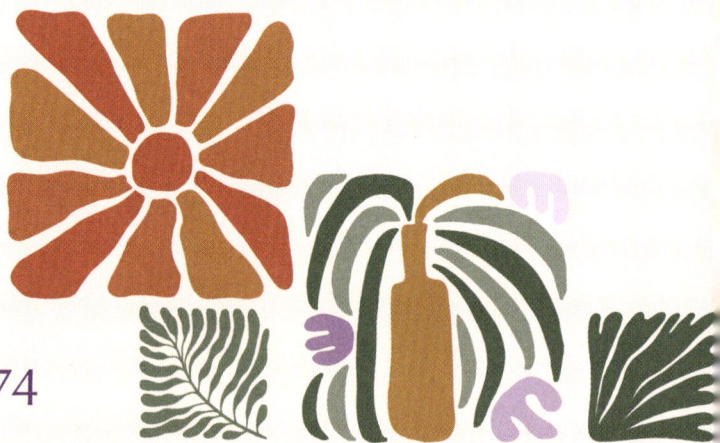

DAY 174
Find Your Rhythm

IDENTIFY THREE TO FIVE DIFFERENT RHYTHMS AND MOVE WITH them. These can be internal rhythms, such as your breath or heartbeat, or sounds from your environment.

DAY 175
Limiting Factors

IDENTIFY FIVE WAYS YOUR CURRENT ENVIRONMENT PREVENTS YOU from connecting to yourself, others, or the world around you.

1. ....
....

2. ....
....

3. ....
....

4. ....
....

5. ....
....

DAY 176
Make Room

DECLUTTER OR ORGANIZE YOUR SPACE. THIS COULD BE YOUR WORK desk, living area, bedroom, or office. Ideally, this is a place you frequent, and when it's messy it influences or reflects your mood or mental capacity.

DAY 177
Connecting to Your Thoughts

PRACTICE CONNECTING TO YOUR BODY THROUGH YOUR MIND. THINK about how you'd like to move and then do it. For example, you might think, *I'm going to wiggle my fingers.* Then wiggle your fingers. Only move as a response to your thoughts.

DAY 178
Connecting to Impulse

ALLOW YOUR BODY TO MOVE IN WHATEVER WAY IT WANTS WITHOUT giving it much thought. Engage in this practice for at least five minutes.

DAY 179
Revisit the Past

IDENTIFY A PAST HOBBY OR INTEREST FROM YOUR CHILDHOOD. Reflect on what you liked about it. What was the reason for letting it go? Do you feel a connection to it as you reminisce? If you find yourself reliving fond memories, give yourself the opportunity to reconnect or reengage with this particular hobby or interest.

DAY 180
How Are You *Moving?*

REFLECT ON YOUR EXPERIENCE PRIORITIZING CONNECTION. IN which areas of your life do you need or want to build connections? Which areas need reinforcement? Which ones feel the strongest?

....

....

....

....

....

....

....

....

....

....

....

....

....

....

....

....

....

....

....

....

....

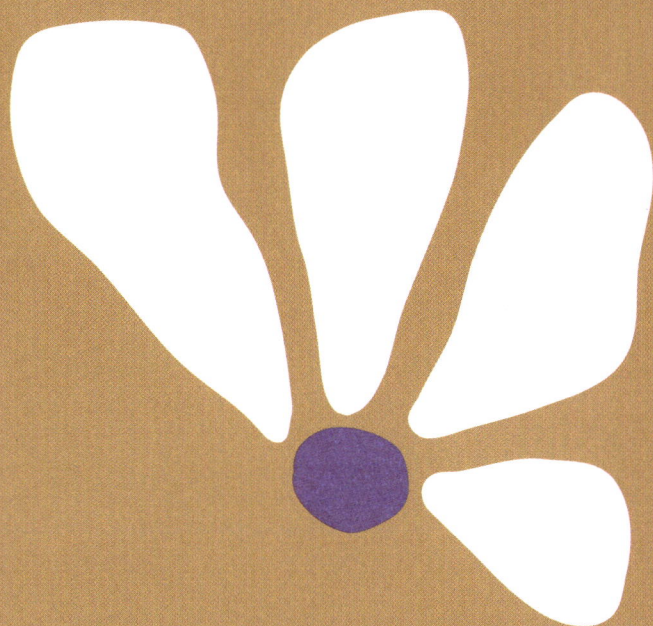

CREATIVE
EXPRESSION
AND PLAY

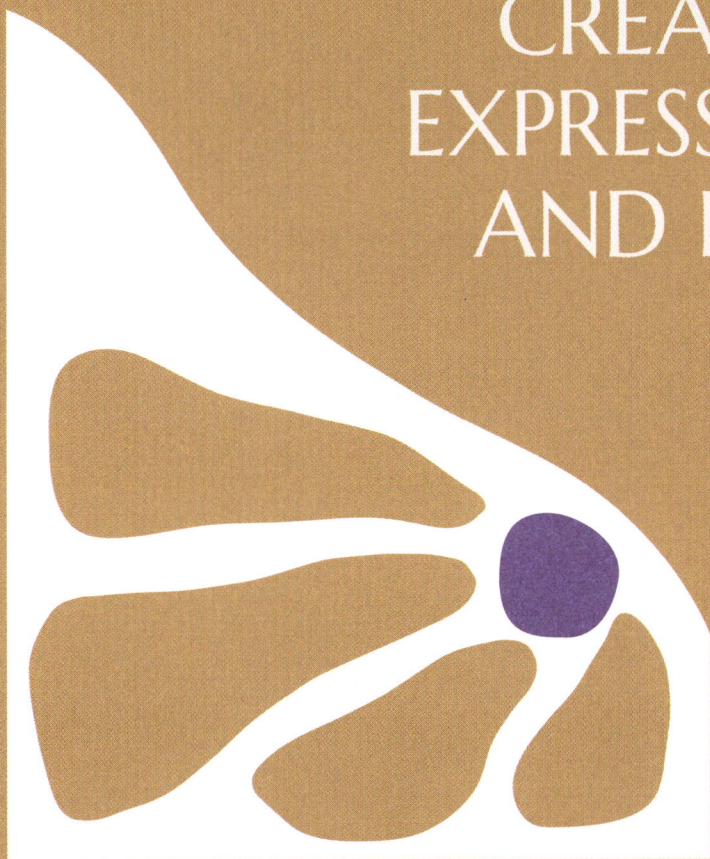

We don't stop playing because we grow old; we grow old because we stop playing.

—George Bernard Shaw

DAY 181
Get Creative

ANY TIME YOU DESIRE TO CHANGE AN ASPECT OF YOURSELF, YOU ARE essentially creating a new version of you. To aid in this change, consider a creative process to get your juices flowing as you embark on the journey. Tapping into your creativity supports regeneration, neuroplasticity, resilience, inner child work, and imagination. Creativity encourages a state of flow that provides stress relief. You might try writing creatively, playing an instrument, drawing or illustrating, coloring, or dancing.

DAY 182
Draw to Music

TURN ON YOUR FAVORITE SONG OR ANY MUSIC AT YOUR DISPOSAL.
Put your pen to paper and do not pick the pen up until the song fin-
ishes. Use the rhythm, tempo, beat, and cadence as a guide for the
movement of your pen.

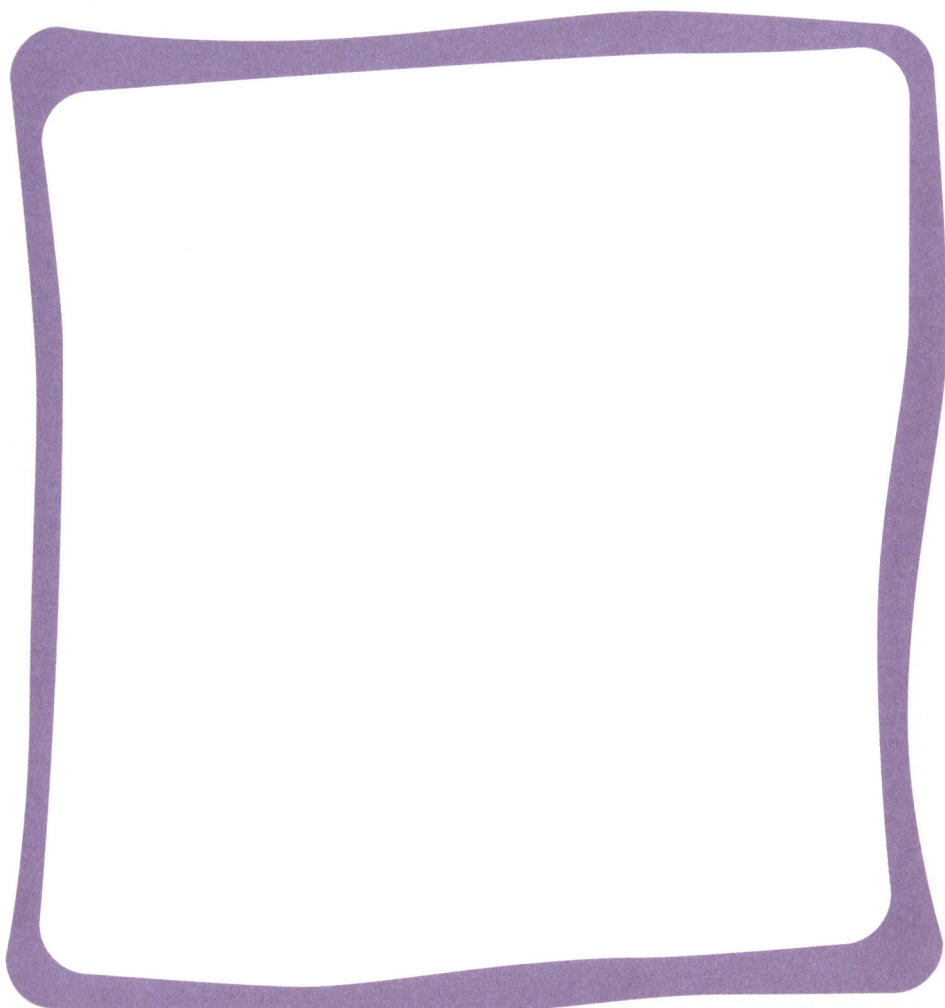

DAY 183
Color

PRINT A FREE COLORING SHEET FROM THE INTERNET, PURCHASE A coloring book, or use a coloring app on a tablet. Allow your imagination to run wild as you color in the pages.

DAY 184
Doodle

Take a pen and a piece of paper and use this space to doodle! Doodling doesn't require any skill. You can make swirls, lines, patterns, and figures. You might even find yourself making notes or doodles in the margins of this book.

DAY 185
Visit a Playground

WHEN WAS THE LAST TIME YOU WENT TO A PLAYGROUND? MOVE-
ments like swinging, hanging, or climbing are so important develop-
mentally, but not just for children. Try on these movements, if you can,
at a local park, school, gym, or even in your own backyard. Many of
these movements, such as climbing a ladder or step stool, can be done
in the comfort of your own home. If you do not have access to these
movements at a playground or in your home, try crawling on the floor,
swinging your arms, or grabbing a doorframe or door handle and leaning or pulling away from it. How does it feel to move in these ways?

DAY 186
Hopscotch

GET SOME CHALK AND CREATE A simple game of hopscotch on a sidewalk or driveway. Embrace the childlike quality of jumping and hopping. When was the last time you played this? How does the jumping and hopping rhythm feel in your body?

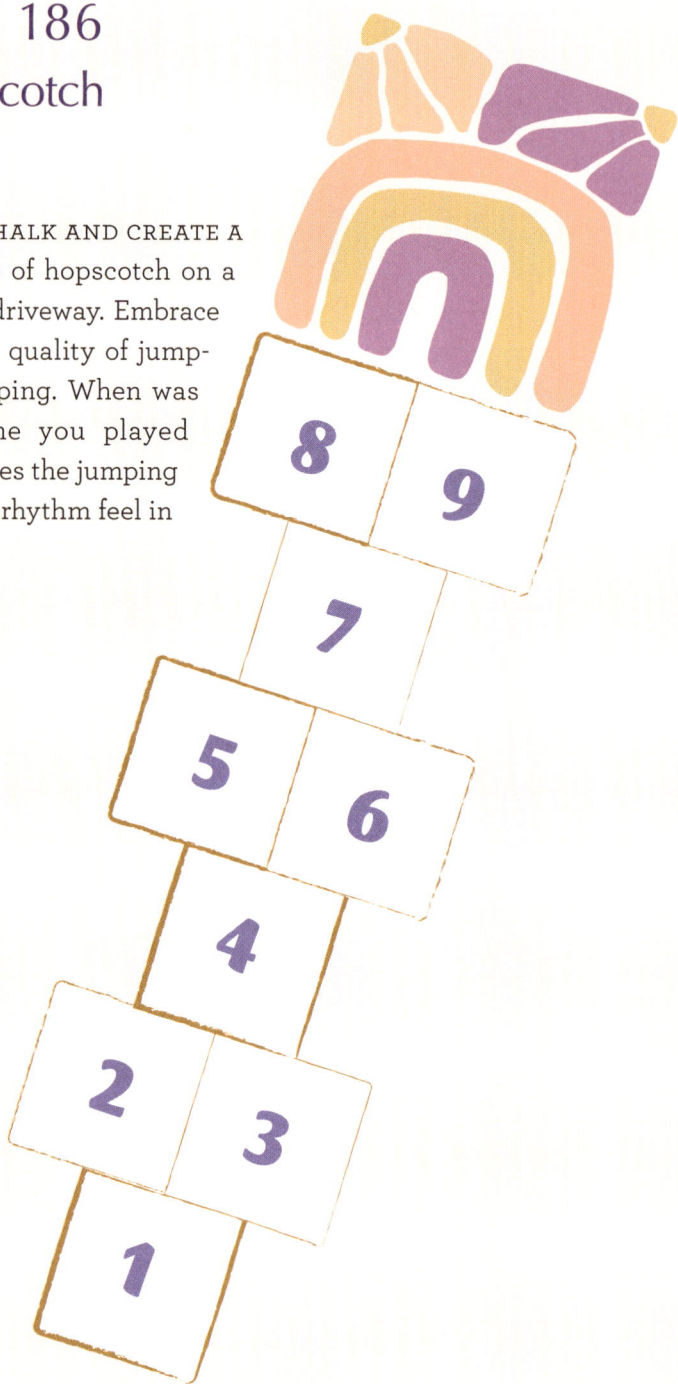

DAY 187
Hop, Skip, Jump

CONTINUING THE EXPERIENCE FROM THE DAY BEFORE, FIND DIFFER-ent ways to explore hopping, jumping, and now skipping in your day. These are all ways to connect to your inner child.

DAY 188
Dress Up

THINK BACK TO WHEN YOU WERE A KID. DID YOU ENJOY PLAYING dress-up? What was your favorite costume or character? Many of us hide behind masks and personas every day. This is an opportunity to show off a part of you, not hide. This can involve wearing a special accessory or outfit or even wearing a costume. Be creative! You don't need a special occasion to dress up. You are the special occasion.

DAY 189
Watch a Movie from Your Youth

THINK OF A MOVIE FROM YOUR YOUTH THAT BRINGS BACK FOND memories. Make time to watch it. Perhaps you might even invite peo-ple you'd like to watch it with.

DAY 190
Read a Book

CURL UP WITH A BOOK, PREFERABLY FICTION. IT DOESN'T HAVE TO BE a long one. Consider reading a book from your childhood. This is an exercise in using your imagination. Turn off the technology, grab a book, and engage your senses as you read, flip pages, and lose yourself in the story.

When was the last time I read this?

....

....

....

How does this story make me feel?

....

....

....

DAY 191
Let It Rain

THE NEXT TIME IT RAINS, GIVE YOURSELF PERMISSION TO DANCE IN the rain, jump in puddles, or walk outside during a gentle storm. Safety is a priority, so this exercise is not to be done in the presence of lightning.

DAY 192
Blow Bubbles

WHETHER IT'S UNDERWATER, using a bubble wand, or into your cup of milk, experience blowing bubbles. This is a wonderful way to support breath, attention, and focus. Plus, it's fun!

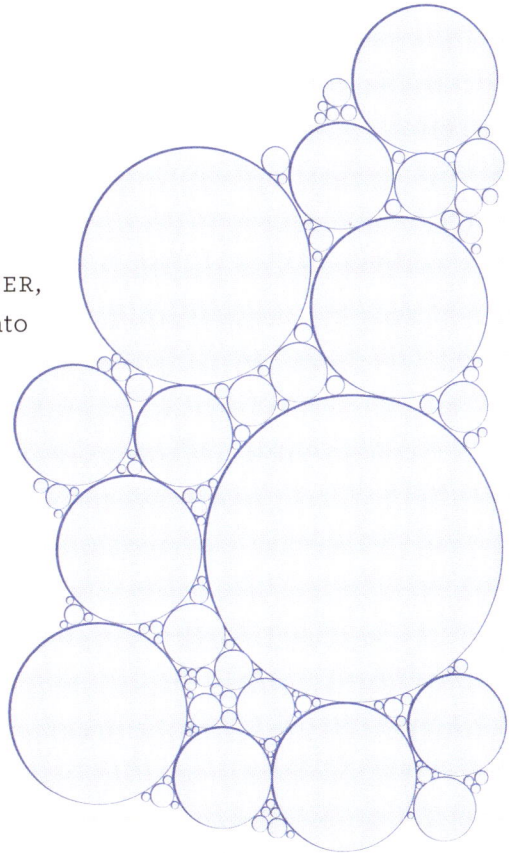

DAY 193
Play with a Child

WHAT BETTER WAY TO EMBRACE YOUR INNER CHILD THAN TO PLAY with a child? Spend time at play with a young person—your own kids, if you have them, or nieces, nephews, and grandchildren. Alternatively, you can volunteer your time to work with kids, babysit, or see a play or improv show put on by children. Embrace the innocent, imaginative world of pretend. Create, explore, and connect to younger movement patterns.

How does this feel for you? Is it difficult to embrace your inner child? What makes this difficult?

....

....

....

....

....

....

....

....

....

....

....

....

....

....

....

DAY 194
Play an Instrument

IF YOU ALREADY PLAY AN INSTRUMENT, THIS IS THE TIME TO INTER-act and practice or improvise. If you do not, this is an opportunity to create and explore sound and rhythm. With permission, pick up a friend's instrument or spend time at a local music store. Sing or make music with household objects.

How does it feel to make music? What is your favorite rhythm or sound?

DAY 195

Lose Yourself to Dance

DANCE IS THE LANGUAGE OF THE SOUL AND SOMETHING WE ALL DO in our youth. Play a favorite song and start moving to the rhythm.

Are you allowed to dance? Is there fear or embarrassment? Is there a need to be "good"? How does it feel when you let go of the judgment and allow your body to move freely?

....

....

....

....

....

....

....

DAY 196
Spend Time in the Garden

PLAY IN THE DIRT OR SAND. PLANT SOME FLOWERS OR SEEDS. THIS IS a big part of childhood. Using your hands, getting down on the ground, and caring for something are great ways to reconnect to your inner child.

DAY 197
Play a Game of Catch

GRAB A BALL AND A FRIEND OR FAMILY MEMBER AND GET TO TOSSing! Can you bring in some playfulness? Play with the distance, height, and speed. Do you feel pressure to catch the ball? Let yourself drop it and see what happens in your body.

DAY 198
Whistle While You Work

CHILDREN ARE FASCINATED WITH THIS SKILL. PERHAPS AS AN ADULT you are still struggling with whistling. That's okay! Practice whistling or attempting to whistle. Pay attention to your lips and the air as it passes through them. Try to whistle a tune or whistle to a song on the radio.

DAY 199
Play a Game

THE POSSIBILITIES HERE ARE ENDLESS. YOU MIGHT TRY A BOARD game, card game, tag, hide-and-seek, and so forth. There is so much benefit to the gentle competition, teamwork, critical thinking, and agility that games require.

DAY 200
Hula-Hoop

WHEN WAS THE LAST TIME YOU USED A HULA-HOOP? YOU MAY HAVE strong feelings around this. Regardless of what they are, get a Hula-Hoop if you can and begin moving. You can use it traditionally around your waist, or if that feels too difficult, use your hands, wrists, or ankles to twirl the hoop. Bring the rhythm into a part of your body. If you do not have access to a Hula-Hoop, exercise your imagination and pretend you are using one. Engage your hips in a circular motion as you attempt to keep the hoop up.

DAY 201
Be Silly

MAKE A SILLY FACE, PLAY A SILLY GAME, OR TRY TO MAKE SOMEONE laugh. This isn't about making sense; it's about sensing.

DAY 202
Walk on the Curb

Pretend the curb is a balance beam and start walking! Use your arms for balance. How far can you go without falling off?

DAY 203
Create a Mandala

ON A BLANK PIECE OF PAPER, DRAW A LARGE CIRCLE. CREATE A design, pattern, or doodle inside the circle. Carl Jung incorporated the ancient symbolic design of mandalas to deepen his patients' awareness of the unconscious. Let your mind go as you engage your fingers in this creative process.

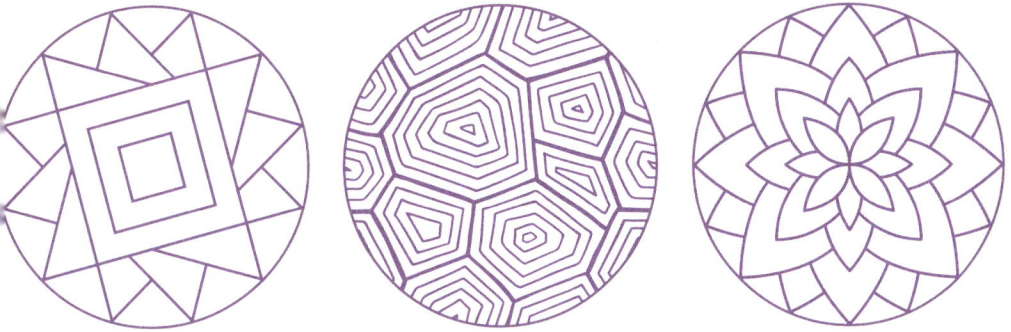

DAY 204
Try a New Movement

EXPLORE AN UNFAMILIAR MOVEMENT PRACTICE, PATTERN, OR rhythm. You can even ask someone to teach you a new movement. Ideally, this is a movement practice contrary in speed or pace to your normal routine. For example, if you always engage in high-intensity exercises, then try Pilates or yoga. Other ideas include swimming, walking, jogging, cooking, painting, and various forms of dance, or you can revisit movement explorations from previous days in this book that were challenging.

DAY 205
Freeze Dance

PLAY A GOOD OLD-FASHIONED GAME OF FREEZE DANCE. THIS requires another person to be in charge of the music and you to be the dancer. Allow yourself to move when the music plays and freeze or pause when the music stops. Can you freeze? How difficult is it to stop and start?

....

....

....

....

....

....

....

....

....

....

....

....

....

....

....

....

DAY 206
The Floor Is Lava

PICK A ROOM IN YOUR HOUSE AND IMAGINE THE FLOOR IS LAVA. YOU
have to get from one side of the room to the other without touching
the floor. You can cover the floor with blankets, towels, or pillows that
are within reach to make it "safely" across the room. Keep in mind
that it isn't the speed at which you cross the room but the strategy
you use to transition from one place to another in a playful and creative manner that is important. Alternatively, you can make objects,
walls, and doors in the room "lava," and rather than avoiding the floor,
maneuver around the room avoiding these objects instead.

DAY 207
Tag!

GRAB SOME FRIENDS OR FAMILY AND PLAY A FRIENDLY GAME OF TAG
or hide-and-seek. The goal here is not to avoid getting found or tagged
but actually to manage the fear of getting caught and the anxiety of
the uncertainty or unknown.

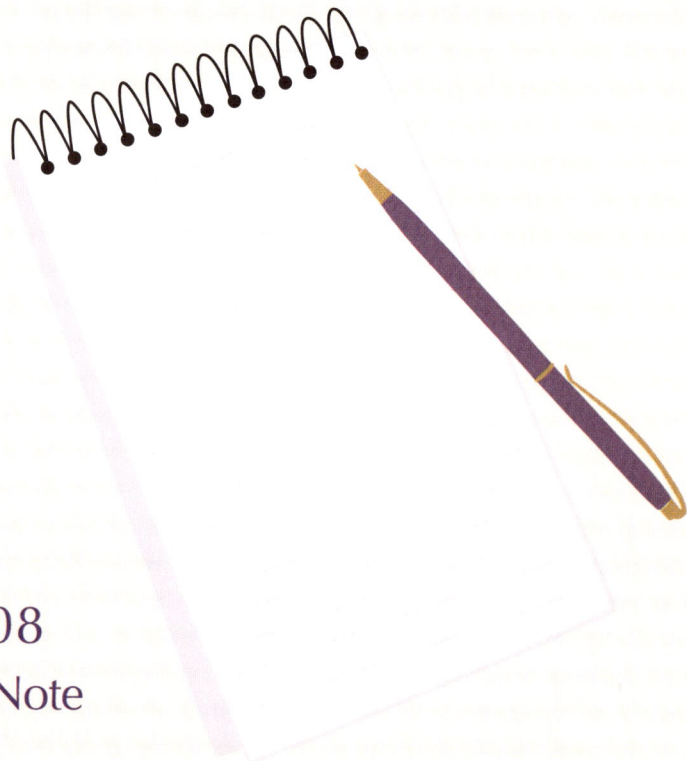

DAY 208
Write a Note

WRITE, DO NOT TEXT, A LITTLE NOTE TO SOMEONE AND GIVE IT TO them. How does it feel to hand it to the person? How does it feel to see their reactions?

DAY 209
Get Messy

THERE'S NO RIGHT WAY TO DO THIS. YOU CAN PAINT, ROLL IN THE dirt, eat with your hands. Can you let yourself get messy without the immediate need to clean up? If you are a parent, how does it feel to let your child get messy? Is there a need to clean it up right away? Can you notice the discomfort? How does this feel in your body?

DAY 210
How Are You *Moving?*

THIS PAST SECTION HAS BEEN ALL ABOUT CONNECTING TO YOUR CRE-
ativity and playfulness. Take time to reflect on how you are moving
through and with your creativity. Which movement qualities are you
engaging in when you are connecting to your inner child?

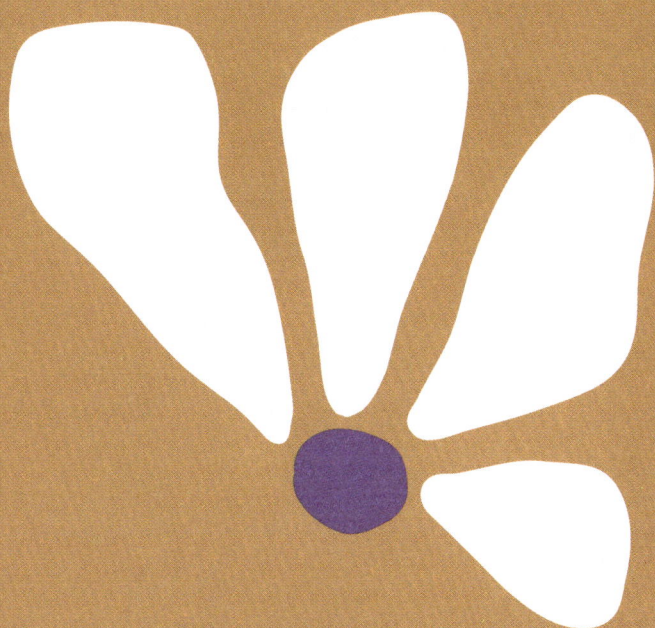

COMMUNICATION

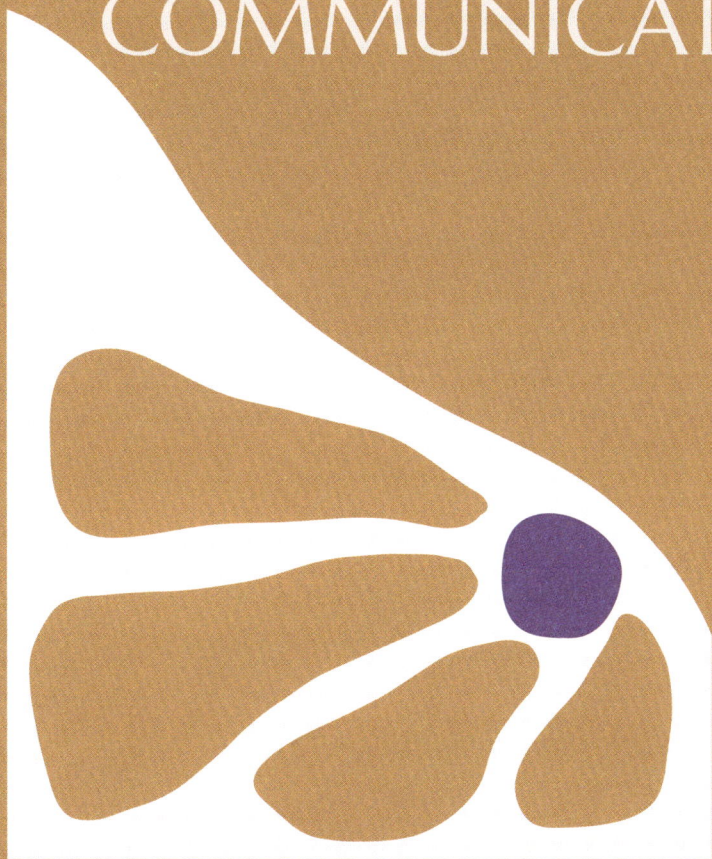

How you communicate with others is an extension of how you talk to yourself. How you speak to yourself is a direct result of how others spoke to you when you were growing up.

DAY 211
How Do You Communicate?

LIST ALL THE WAYS YOU COMMUNICATE. THIS SHOULD INCLUDE VERbal and nonverbal methods. For example, texting, emailing, speaking, writing, gesturing. What are your preferred methods of communication? What might be lost in translation?

....

....

....

....

....

DAY 212
Exploring Communication

WHAT DO YOU BELIEVE TO BE UNHEALTHY COMMUNICATION? WHAT does healthy communication look or feel like? With whom do you have healthy communication? With whom would you like to have healthy communication?

....

....

....

....

....

DAY 213
Misunderstandings

IMAGINE A TIME WHEN YOU OR YOUR INTENTIONS WERE MISUNDER-
stood. How does it feel to be misunderstood? How do you feel when
you misunderstand someone else? What happens in your body when
you feel misunderstood?

....

....

....

....

....

....

....

....

....

....

....

DAY 214
Patterns of Communication

IDENTIFY YOUR PATTERNS OF COMMUNICATION. ARE YOU DIRECT with your communication? Do you beat around the bush or have difficulty expressing what you need? Do you ask for help?

Now consider how your patterns of communication affect your movement behaviors. Bring into awareness your comfort level with eye contact, body language, and active listening. How does your body show up during these patterns of communication?

....

....

....

....

....

....

....

....

....

....

DAY 215
Conflict

BRING TO MIND A TIME WHEN YOU FELT CONFLICTED. HOW DO YOU feel about conflict? Where do you feel it in your body? What does your body need to resolve or to move through the conflict?

....

....

....

....

....

....

....

....

....

....

DAY 216
Skirting the Issue

PLACE AN OBJECT ON THE GROUND IN FRONT OF YOU. MOVE IN A WAY that forces you to avoid the object. Now imagine this object is an issue, conflict, or need. How does it feel to avoid this? How does your body react and feel during this exercise?

....

....

....

....

....

....

....

....

....

....

DAY 217
Direct Communication

THIS EXERCISE IS A PRACTICE IN IDENTIFYING YOUR NEEDS AND embodying how to communicate succinctly and in a straightforward manner. Make a list of needs or desires—for example, "I need a raise," "I need assistance," or "I need your support."

....

....

....

....

....

Next, either take your index finger and tap the air in front of you as if dotting an *i* or place your hands about three inches apart with your palms facing each other. Integrate a need or desire with the gesture. This allows each statement to have structure, focus, and intensity in a way that supports direct communication.

DAY 218
Take Your Time Responding

When you are responding to a text, an email, or a phone call, take a full breath or two after reading or hearing the message before responding. This creates space between your reaction and your action to respond, allowing you to decide instead of react.

DAY 219
Don't Respond

No response is still a response. Not everything needs to be responded to. Practice holding off on a response to a social call, email, or text that is not urgent or time sensitive. It can be challenging to decipher what is urgent and what is perceived as urgent, especially when everything feels urgent in today's communication.

Notice how it feels or what comes up in your mind when you do not respond. Is the person expecting a response? Is there pressure or expectation to respond in a timely manner?

Practice physically stabilizing your body to support connection and grounding in the moment.

DAY 220
Hello

FIND THREE WAYS TO SAY "HELLO" WITHOUT WORDS. PRACTICE COM-municating in this way. Identify other actions you can say without words and practice those at your leisure. Examples are "goodbye," "I love you," and "no."

Reflect on how it feels to engage in this exercise.

....

....

....

....

....

....

....

....

....

....

DAY 221
Talk with Your Hands

RESEARCH SHOWS THAT USING YOUR HANDS WHEN YOU SPEAK increases your connection to your own imagination and creativity. Practice using your hands to support your verbal communication. What is the most interesting part of this experience? Is this familiar or unfamiliar?

....

....

....

....

....

....

....

....

....

....

DAY 222
Belly Button

STUDIES INDICATE THAT THE DIRECTION YOUR BELLY BUTTON IS FAC-ing correlates with your area of focus, attraction, or attention. Bring attention to your navel region, a.k.a. your belly button. Become aware of the direction it is currently facing. Where is your attention or attraction currently focused? With regard to communication, make an effort to communicate by facing your belly button toward the person with whom you are speaking.

DAY 223
Listen with Your Body, Not Just Your Ears

YOU CAN LISTEN WITH MORE THAN JUST YOUR EARS. EMPATHIC LIS-tening involves connecting with someone's body, not just the words coming out of their mouth. Notice the person's body language, tone, and spatial plane. Find ways to match their posture, volume, and phys-ical level, and ensure that you can physically see eye to eye.

DAY 224
Ghosting

BRING TO MIND A TIME WHEN SOMEONE, WITHOUT ANY REASON OR explanation, stopped communicating with you. Ghosting is different from boundary setting, when someone says, "I need time and will reach out when I'm ready." In the ghosting scenario, the other person simply ends all contact.

How did this feel? What is the hardest part? What do you want versus need in this situation?

....

....

....

....

DAY 225
Self-Reflection

PRACTICE EXPRESSING DIFFERENT EMOTIONS IN THE MIRROR. CAN you exaggerate or play with them?

How do your facial features express certain emotions? How does it feel to witness your own emotions? Is it difficult? How so?

....

....

....

....

DAY 226
Talk to a Stranger

STRIKE UP A CONVERSATION WITH A STRANGER: THE BARISTA AT THE coffee shop, a sales associate, or the person standing next to you in line. After, reflect on how it felt to talk to someone you don't know, or how it felt if they were not receptive or open to dialogue. What was happening in your body as the experience unfolded?

....

....

....

....

....

....

....

....

....

....

....

....

....

....

....

....

....

....

DAY 227
"I Feel . . ."

EVERY DAY IS AN OPPORTUNITY TO COMMUNICATE HOW AND WHAT you feel. Practice verbally expressing how you feel by saying something to yourself or out loud to someone else. There is so much benefit to acknowledging and validating your emotions. Notice what is happening in your body when you name the feeling or emotion. Become aware of how your body is expressing this feeling you have identified.

DAY 228
Call Someone

INTENTIONALLY CALL SOMEONE ON THE PHONE AND have a conversation. Do not FaceTime or video chat with the person. This exercise is specifically about hearing and talking, not seeing. Is this a familiar sensation? How does it feel to talk on the phone as opposed to texting or FaceTiming?

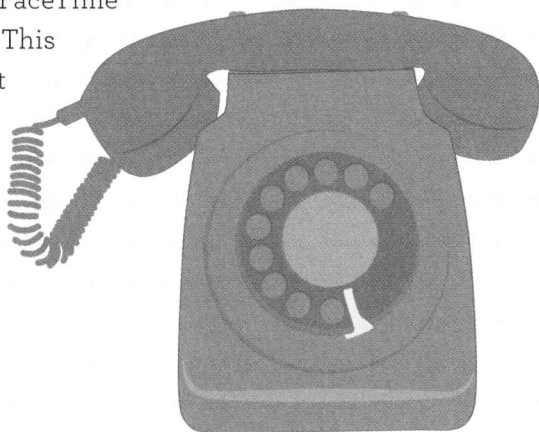

DAY 229
Play a Game of Charades

CHARADES IS A GREAT WAY TO CONVEY A THOUGHT OR TO COMMUNI-cate an idea without words. You do not have to start a formal game. Perhaps during your next get together, create topics or themes or just pick ideas off the top of your head. This is not a practice in winning but in communicating.

DAY 230
See Something, Say Something

YOU MAY FIND IT DIFFICULT TO KNOW WHEN TO SAY SOMETHING. This is an exercise in communicating what you see. Keep in mind that this does not have to be something urgent or threatening. It can be noticing the sunshine, weather, someone's aesthetic, or a feeling about a present situation. Also keep in mind that this is not a practice in harming or offending but in expressing what you observe, naming what you see, and communicating effectively.

DAY 231
Speak Up, Speak Out

WHEN YOU SPEAK, YOUR TONE OF VOICE IS SOMETIMES MORE IMPOR-
tant than the specific words you use. Bring awareness to *how* you say
whatever you say. Notice the inflection and intonation as well as the
volume. Play with the volume, speed, rhythm, and cadence of the
words you speak. You can practice matching the volume and tone of
the person with whom you are communicating.

Are certain tones or volumes more difficult for me than
others? Why?

....

....

....

....

....

....

....

DAY 232
Write It Down to Talk It Out

TALKING MAY BE DIFFICULT, ESPECIALLY IN A CHALLENGING CON-
versation. Practice writing down what you want to say beforehand.
This helps provide steadiness and readiness in the face of discomfort,
fear, trepidation, or anxiety.

DAY 233
Lean In to Conflict

CONFLICT CAN COME WITH TENSION AND DISCOMFORT. YOU MAY BE inclined to avoid or run away from conflict; however, leaning in to conflict, naming it, and identifying how you feel as it comes up are powerful ways to show up and move through the friction.

Identify a current conflict or instance that creates conflict and notice how your body responds. Rather than dismissing, avoiding, or ignoring it, find ways to interact with the sensation as it arises in your body. Is there a pressure or weight to it? Move with it.

....

....

....

....

....

DAY 234
Stand Up for Yourself

BECOME AWARE OF HOW YOUR BODY MOVES WHEN IT ENCOUNTERS conflict or tension. Plant your feet and find your vertical. Imagine your feet are the roots of your tree. Feel the energy from the floor move through your body and out the crown of your head as you lengthen your spine.

DAY 235
Identify Your Needs

IDENTIFY A NEED IN THE FACE OF CONFLICT. HOW CAN YOU ASK FOR
what you need? Perhaps this is something you can do for yourself.
If not, identify the support you need and ask for it. An easy way to
practice this is when you order food. What would it look like to ask for
exactly what you want without making excuses or minimizing your
needs?

*What makes it hard for me to ask for something, espe-
cially during times of conflict?*

....
....
....

Do I have difficulty receiving support or assistance?

....
....
....

What does my body need to accept help?

....
....
....

DAY 236
Take Responsibility

RESPONSIBILITY REQUIRES A RESPONSE, NOT A REACTION. REVISIT
the section on regulation (starting with Day 61). Find ways to regulate
your reaction during a conflict. When you feel more grounded and
responsive, identify your role in this conflict. Take responsibility for
your reaction or feelings in this moment by naming them or letting the
person you are experiencing conflict with know. Be aware of whether
you feel responsible for the other person's feelings or reactions.

Is it difficult for me to take responsibility?

....
....
....

Is it easy for me to take responsibility for others' emo-
tions? How long has that been a pattern? Where did I
learn that?

....
....
....

DAY 237
Don't Apologize

IF YOU ARE SOMEONE WHO APOLOGIZES FOR EVERYTHING, EVEN when you did nothing wrong, this exercise may be challenging. It requires you to recognize not only when to offer an apology but also when *not* to apologize.

Think of the phrase "I'm sorry." What do you notice in your body when you speak it? What does this tell you about how you respond in times of conflict?

An apology is an opportunity for reflection and taking responsibility. Consider where you feel remorse or guilt in your body. The presence of these sensations can guide you toward repair in acknowledging your role in the conflict. This can also make space for validating how you feel wronged and identifying what you feel needs repair.

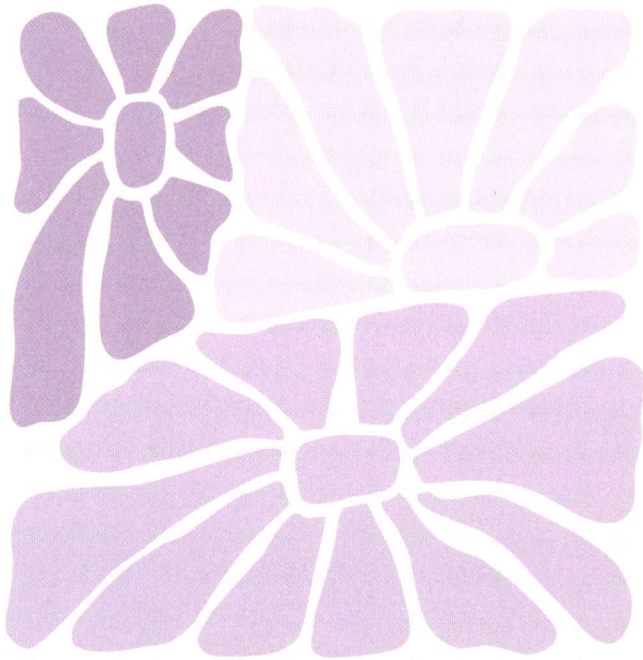

DAY 238
Voice Your Ideas

WHEN ASKED, "WHAT DO YOU WANT TO DO?" HAVE YOU EVER responded with "I don't care" or "Whatever you want"? Often we respond like this to appear accommodating, to avoid conflict, or to people-please and mitigate others disliking us.

Become aware of what happens in your body with this question and challenge it. For example, you may notice your shoulders shrug, you shake your head, or you drop your gaze. Find ways to shift your movement to reinforce your willingness and ability to offer a suggestion or idea. This is another opportunity to communicate a desire or need.

DAY 239
An Attitude of Gratitude

EVERYONE WANTS TO FEEL APPRECIATED. WHEN YOU PRACTICE PUT-
ting gratitude out into the world, it gets returned. Identify things you
are grateful for or appreciative of. Connect to your sensation of gratitude. Where does your body feel gratitude, and how does it show
appreciation? If this involves other people, find a way to communicate
this to them.

DAY 240
How Are You *Moving?*

TAKE SOME TIME TO REFLECT ON THE EXERCISES IN THIS LAST SEC-
tion on communication. What have you learned about your movement
patterns that either hinder or facilitate communication?

Reflect on what you need to prioritize to foster healthy communication.

....

....

....

....

....

....

....

....

....

....

....

....

....

....

....

....

....

....

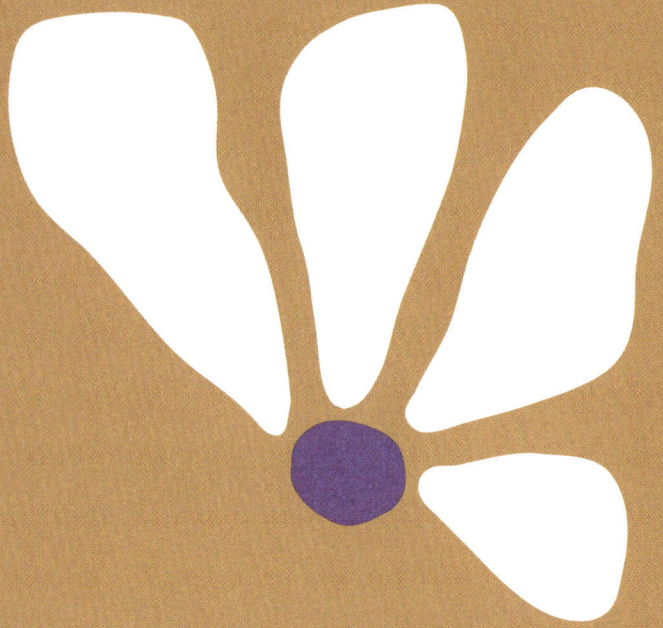

BOUNDARIES

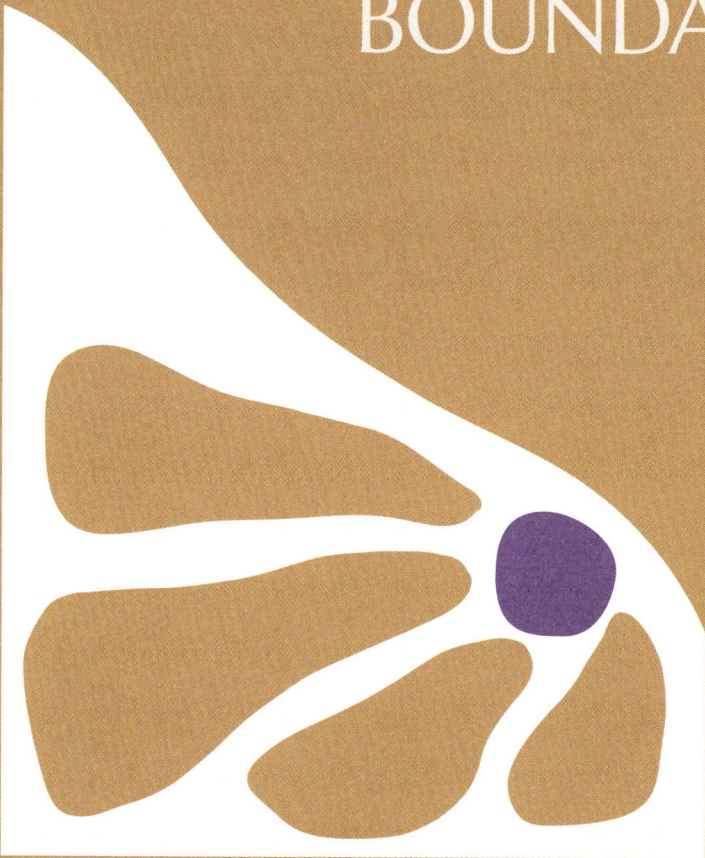

Boundaries do not come from rigidity. They come from flexibility of mind and body.

DAY 241
Reflecting on Boundaries

LET'S LOOK AT YOUR CURRENT RELATIONSHIP WITH BOUNDARIES. Reflect on the following:

Do I have difficulty setting boundaries?

....

....

Do I have difficulty receiving or hearing a boundary?

....

....

Who modeled my current relationship with boundaries?

....

....

Why do I feel boundaries are needed?

....

....

DAY 242
Boundaries / No Boundaries

DRAW A VERTICAL LINE IN THE SPACE BELOW. ON ONE SIDE OF THE line, write BOUNDARIES at the top, and on the other side, write NO BOUNDARIES. Draw what each looks like for you. You can express using abstract images, lines, or shapes or draw a detailed scene. Allow what each state feels like to dictate what you draw. For example, if boundaries feel rigid and confining, create images that illustrate those feelings.

DAY 243
Request Versus Boundary

A REQUEST REQUIRES SOMEONE ELSE TO CHANGE THEIR BEHAVIOR, whereas a boundary requires you to change your behavior.

Request: "Lower your voice."

Boundary: "I will not continue this conversation if you yell at me."

Identify requests you have made and boundaries you'd like to set. Reflect on the following questions as you revisit them.

How do I move when making a request? What gestures or postures are present?

....

....

....

How do I move when setting a boundary? What gestures or postures are present or absent?

....

....

....

DAY 244
Embodying Boundaries

REVISIT YOUR DRAWINGS FROM DAY 242. CREATE A MOVEMENT, POS-
ture, or gesture that represents the overall theme of each side. What
does it look like to embody your boundaries? What does it look like
to have no boundaries? Bring into your body the qualities of each—
the shape, speed, and space of the movement. What do you notice in
each movement experience? What stands out to you as you move your
boundaries or lack thereof?

....

....

....

....

....

....

....

....

....

....

....

....

....

....

....

....

DAY 245
Either/Or

BOUNDARIES ARE OFTEN PERCEIVED AS ALL OR NOTHING, LACKING flexibility. Let's explore this polarization.

Take two minutes to explore the physical sensations of rigidity. Rigidity may feel like $x, y, z \ldots$

....

....

....

Take two minutes to explore the physical sensations of fluidity. Fluidity may feel like $a, b, c \ldots$

....

....

....

DAY 246
From One End to Another

Deepening the exploration from Day 245, create a scale of your living space. One end of the room is rigidity, and the other end is fluidity.

RIGIDITY–FLUIDITY

Travel between the two and notice how they are connected rather than separate. Identify where you feel most comfortable on this scale and engage in this movement for two or three minutes.

DAY 247
"No."

EMBODY YOUR "NO."

How does my "no" move?

....

....

....

How do I move when I am told "no"?

....

....

....

DAY 248
"Yes."

EMBODY YOUR "YES."

How do I move when I say "yes"?

....
....
....

How do I move when someone says "yes"?

....
....
....

DAY 249
Move "Maybe"

SAY "MAYBE" OUT LOUD AND NOTICE WHAT YOUR BODY DOES. HOW does your facial expression change? Do your shoulders move? Does your torso or chest shift in any way?

Once you identify the movement signature of your "maybe," exaggerate it.

Reflect on how it feels when you are in your "maybe."

Is there a "no" really wanting to emerge?

....
....
....

Is there pressure to make a decision?

....
....
....

What do I need in order to sit in the discomfort of indecision?

....
....
....

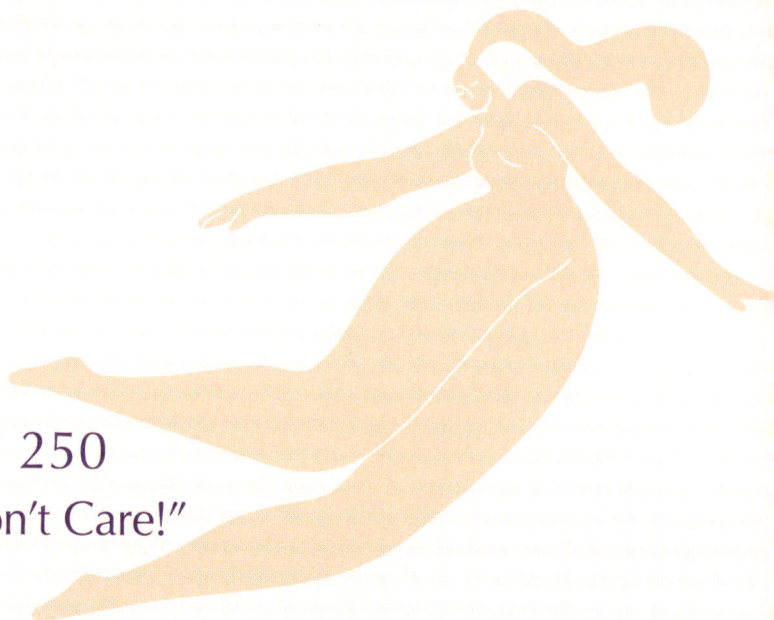

DAY 250
"I Don't Care!"

CONSIDER YOUR RESPONSE WHEN SOMEONE ASKS FOR YOUR OPINION. Perhaps you often respond with "Whatever." Ask yourself, *Do I have an opinion, or am I just trying to make the other person feel comfortable or in charge? Am I simply wanting the other person to like me?*

Take a moment to try on your "I don't care." Does your body shrink? Is there any tension? What is underneath it? This can help clarify and direct what you really need or want.

DAY 251
"Stop."

SAY "STOP" OUT LOUD AND NOTICE WHAT YOUR BODY DOES IN response. Repeat the word a few times and allow your body to move in accordance.

How does my body communicate when it has had enough or needs a break?

....

....

....

Do I have difficulty stopping? Why?

....

....

....

DAY 252
Push It

BRING TO MIND A MOMENT WHEN SOMEONE PUSHED YOU AROUND, enforced their agenda, or tried to coerce you into a decision you weren't ready to make.

How does it feel to be pushed around? What happens to your movement?

....

....

....

....

....

....

....

....

....

....

DAY 253
Push Over

YOU MAY BE FAMILIAR WITH THE WORD *PUSHOVER*. PHYSICALLY allow your body to try on being "pushed over."

What is the most striking part of this?

....

....

....

What is missing from my movement?

....

....

....

What do I need in order to not be pushed over?

....

....

....

DAY 254
Bend Over

WHEN SOMEONE IS A PEOPLE PLEASER, THERE IS OFTEN AN ASSOCIA-
tion with bending over backward. Without causing harm or injury,
imagine or try bending backward. Consider that boundaries come
from flexibility, not rigidity. However, too much flexibility, meaning
hyperextension, can put us physically and emotionally out.

Practice bending over (forward or backward) in a way that challenges your flexibility while not compromising or sacrificing your self.

DAY 255

Stand Your Ground

PLANT YOUR FEET ON THE GROUND WHILE KEEPING A SLIGHT BEND
in your knees. Widen your stance and find the optimal position that
allows you to maintain a connection with your center of gravity and
the ground. You can play with opening your stance too wide and
standing with your feet too close together to gauge the position you
feel sturdiest in, where you can maintain your balance and posture.
Try placing one foot slightly in front of the other to create an even
sturdier base. Notice which foot feels more secure in front. This is
your decision pose.

DAY 256
Identify Your Boundaries

BOUNDARIES CAN BE SEEN AS BORDERS. LET'S EXPLORE YOUR PHYSI-cal boundaries. With one hand, trace your body with your palm, from the top of your head down to your feet. Apply a bit of pressure when needed and be sure to trace as much of your body as possible: every curve, indentation, and protrusion. Notice where your physical boundaries end and where the air around you begins.

DAY 257
Push into the Wall

BOUNDARIES ARE AN EXPLORATION OF where you end and another person or thing begins. Place your hands shoulder width apart on the wall and push. What do you notice in your body and mind as you apply pressure? Try pushing away and leaning in. Which one feels more familiar? Notice as you step away from the wall how your body feels.

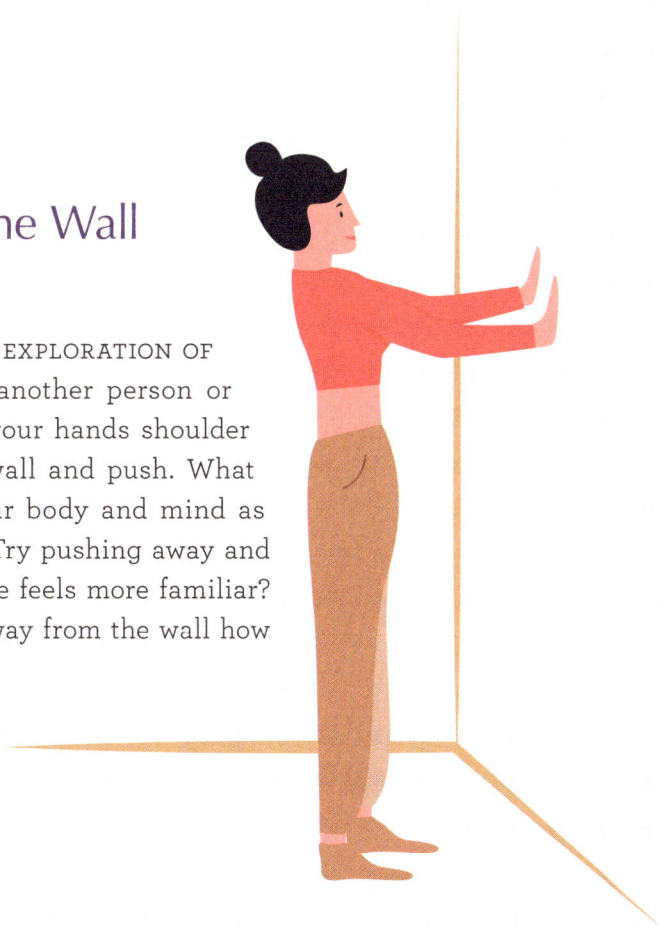

DAY 258
Got Your Back

Sit or stand with your back against the wall. Allow the wall to support you. Lean or push into the wall and pay attention to what happens in your body and mind as you feel supported in this way. How does this differ from the sensation in the previous exercise?

DAY 259
Maintain Your Distance

Stand inside a boundary, such as a circle, box, or border. You can create a boundary by standing inside a Hula-Hoop, a rope, or a scarf or towel spread on the floor. Ask a trusted individual with whom you have good rapport to walk toward the boundary in front of you. Notice how your body alerts you when this person gets too close for comfort. If it feels possible, do this with the person approaching from behind you and allow your body to move or respond as needed to support safety and mitigate perceived threat in the moment.

DAY 260
Scapular Push-Ups

BOUNDARIES COME FROM AWARENESS OF THE SHOULDER BLADES. Place your hands shoulder width apart on the wall. With your arms straight (but elbows not locked), allow your upper back to relax and draw your shoulder blades together, imagining them touching. Draw your shoulder blades down your back and push away from the wall. The motion resembles that of a push-up, but the movement is isolated to the shoulder blades.

DAY 261
Near Space

EXPLORE THE SPACE CLOSE TO YOUR BODY. KEEP IN MIND THAT YOUR movements will be smaller as you explore the area directly around your body. How does it feel to stay or play small? How familiar is this sensation? Is there an urge to expand or move away from your body?

....

....

....

....

DAY 262

Far Space

ALLOW YOUR BODY TO EXTEND OR REACH INTO THE SPACE AROUND you. Take up as much space as you feel safe doing. Engage in large, indulgent movements. How does it feel to move in this way? How does it compare to the previous exercise of playing small?

....

....

....

....

DAY 263
Follow-the-Leader

EMPLOY THE ASSISTANCE OF A TRUSTED FRIEND OR FAMILY MEMBER. Invite them to play a game of follow-the-leader. Take turns leading and following. Here are some rules when playing the game:

- Do not mock or mimic each other.
- Do not attempt to trick or confuse the other person.
- Identify a "safe word" that lets each of you know it's time to switch or you need a break.

See whether there is a difference between mirroring, or facing each other, and being in front of each other.

Which feels more familiar? Which did you prefer? What does this say with regard to your ability to lead or follow in your professional and personal life?

....

....

....

....

....

....

....

....

....

....

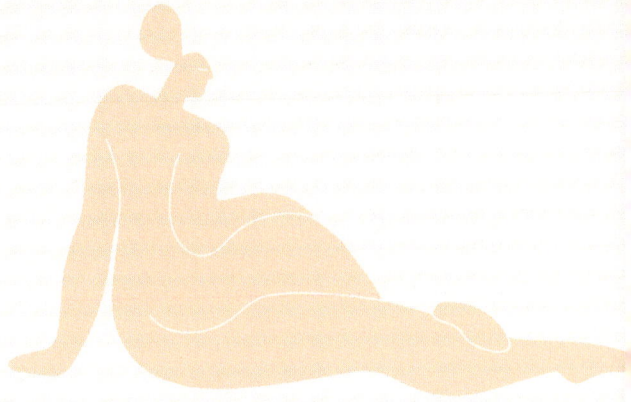

DAY 264
Move a Body Part in As Many Ways As Possible

HEALTHY BOUNDARIES ARE MORE A REFLECTION OF FLEXIBILITY than rigidity. Isolate a part of your body and move it in as many ways as safely possible. Move on to other body parts that you feel called to explore.

Which parts feel more flexible than others? What did you find difficult about this exercise?

....
....
....
....
....
....
....
....
....
....

DAY 265
Less Is More

THIS IS AN EXERCISE IN SIMPLIFICATION. IDENTIFY A PHYSICAL activity or current movement and see how simple you can make it. Break it down into steps. Slow the movement down. Let go of an unnecessary tension. Notice where you are holding or bracing. Remember to breathe into the movement.

Reflect on this exercise.

Do I consider myself a multitasker? What do I notice about my overall productivity when attempting to do multiple things at once?

....

....

What happens to the quality of my productivity when I slow down and focus on one thing at a time?

....

....

Do I find it hard to slow down? How much is my productivity tied to speed and pace?

....

....

DAY 266
Slow Your Response

NOTICE YOUR EAGERNESS TO SAY "YES" OR "NO." BECOME AWARE OF the trajectory of your movement or body posture in those moments. Assuming your body is leaning forward even slightly, find your way back to a vertical posture before deciding and responding.

DAY 267
Power of Pause

THIS IS ANOTHER EXERCISE IN RESPONSE TIME. ANY TIME YOU notice pressure building in your body over responding to someone's inquiry, take a full breath cycle before responding. The most important part of this is the exhale. Make sure that you allow for the air to fully leave your lungs before you respond to the question.

How often do I feel pressured to respond? How does this affect my ability to manage my expectations and self-care?

....

....

....

....

....

....

....

....

....

....

....

....

....

....

....

....

DAY 268
Embrace the Small Decisions

You make decisions every day, many of which go unnoticed. Draw your attention to the small or even unconscious decisions you make, such as during your morning routine, commute, or interactions with your family.

Which decisions do I take for granted? How does it feel to make a decision? Do I notice a sense of accomplishment?

....

....

....

....

....

....

....

....

....

....

....

....

....

....

....

....

....

....

DAY 269
Honor Your Boundaries

MAKE A LIST OF BOUNDARIES THAT YOU ALREADY PRIORITIZE. Reflect on how it feels to honor these and what happened and how it felt when you did not.

....

....

....

....

....

Now make a list of the boundaries you want to prioritize. What do you need to do to prioritize them?

....

....

....

....

....

DAY 270
How Are You *Moving*?

WHAT ARE YOUR TAKEAWAYS FROM THIS SECTION? HOW ARE YOU feeling physically and emotionally about boundaries? How has your body's relationship to boundaries changed over the last thirty days?

....
....
....
....
....
....
....
....
....
....
....
....
....
....
....
....
....

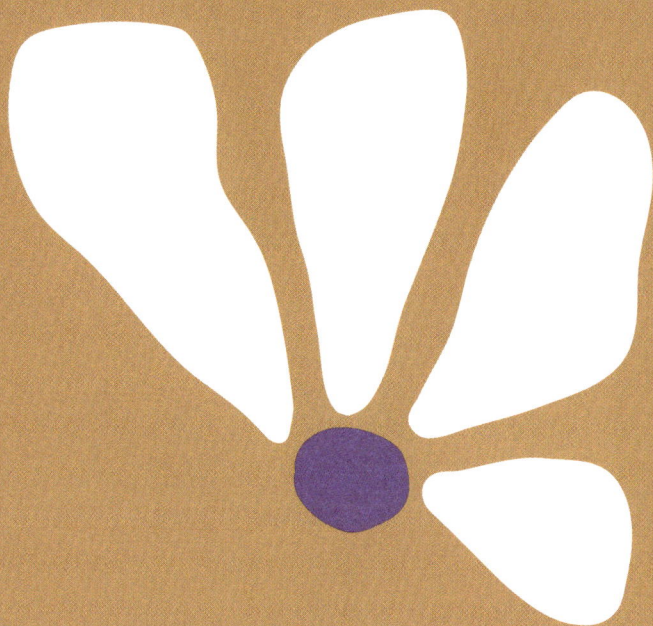

TRUST

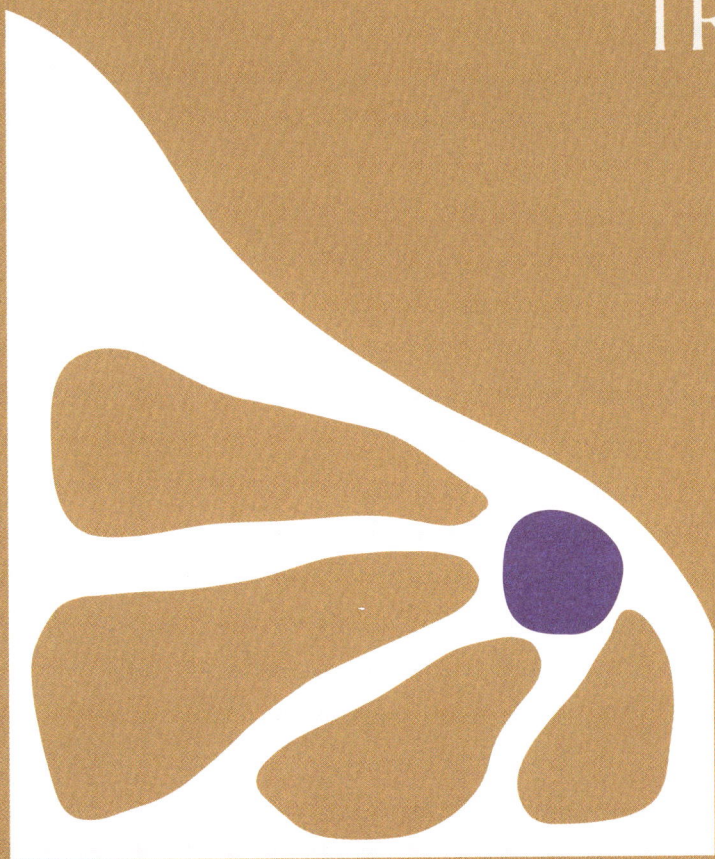

You cannot trust a body
you hate or fear.

DAY 271
Feel Trust

WHAT DOES TRUST FEEL LIKE IN YOUR BODY? SIT WITH THE WORD *trust* in your mind. What sensations do you notice in your body? What is your current relationship with trust? How do you know when you trust someone? Whom do you trust? Do you trust yourself?

....

....

....

....

....

....

....

....

....

....

DAY 272
Gut Reaction

PEOPLE OFTEN REFER TO A *GUT REACTION* WHEN THEY ARE FOLLOW-
ing their instincts. Our gut can be a tricky place, especially if you
feel your anxiety or fear there, as many people do. This exercise is
about deciphering the different sensations and signals in your body.
What would it look like to "trust your gut" instead of focusing on
your gut reaction?

....

....

....

....

....

....

....

....

....

....

DAY 273
Intuition

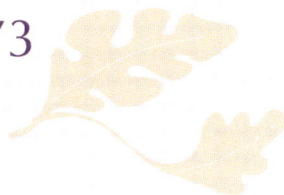

INTUITION IS A SENSE THAT HELPS US TAP INTO OUR SELF-TRUST. This exercise is about connecting to your intuition. The three centers of your intuition are your head, heart, and belly (just under the navel). Bring awareness to these body parts by placing a hand gently on each. By simultaneously placing both hands on these parts of your body, you can intentionally connect to your intuition centers.

DAY 274

Doubt It

SHRUGGING IS ONE WAY YOUR BODY MAY EXUDE OR SUGGEST DOUBT. Your shoulders may be signaling when you doubt your own words or feelings. Pay attention to times when you say something that you aren't sure you agree with. Practice shrugging one shoulder at a time and both shoulders simultaneously to become more familiar with this sensation.

DAY 275
Likes Versus Dislikes

TAKE A MOMENT TO LIST WHAT YOU KNOW YOU LIKE AND WHAT YOU know you do not, such as foods, hobbies, sports, movies, people, jobs, or chores.

....
....
....
....
....
....
....
....
....
....
....
....
....
....
....
....
....
....
....
....
....

DAY 276
Trust Your Timing

FIND A PLACE WHERE YOU CAN WALK AROUND WITHOUT ANY OBSTA-cles in your way. Begin walking at a brisk pace. Play with the speed of your walk and find the pace that feels right for you. Trust your body to guide you to find the speed at which you can notice your surroundings and have internal awareness as well.

DAY 277

Walk Backward

ONCE AGAIN, FIND A PLACE WHERE YOU CAN WALK WITHOUT ANY obstacles in your way. Begin walking backward. Become aware of how this feels and how comfortable you are moving from your back space. Do you trust yourself as you walk backward?

DAY 278
Move from Mind

Think about how you want to move and then do it. Become aware of the connection between mind and body and the interplay between them. Does your mind trust what your body can do?

DAY 279
Move from Body

Allow your body to move improvisationally however it wants. Become aware of how much your mind wants to take over or lead the way. Can your mind trust that your body knows what it needs without judgment or interference?

DAY 280
Body Trust

TAKE A MOMENT TO IDENTIFY WHAT your body needs. Notice what signals and sensations are present. Perhaps you are thirsty, hungry, or need to use the bathroom. Are you uncomfortable or feeling insecure in your surroundings? Trust that your body knows what it needs and practice honoring its needs.

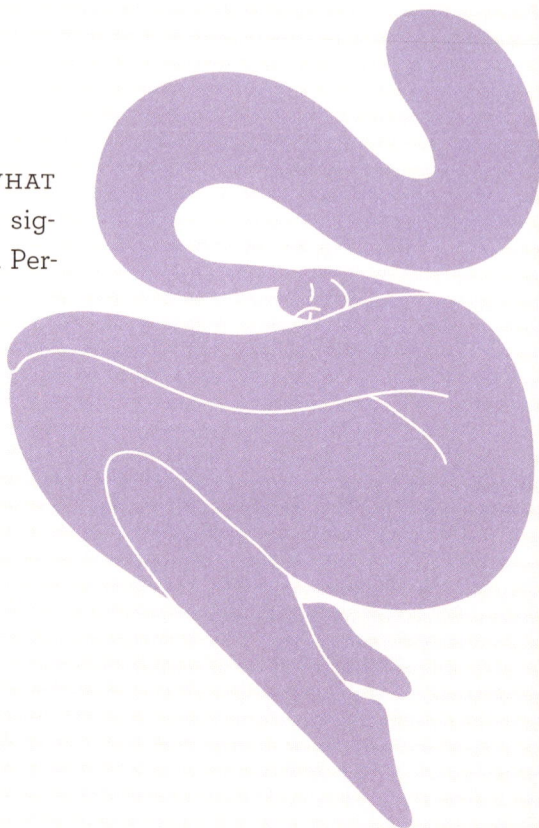

DAY 281
Brace Yourself

YOU MAY FIND THAT YOUR BODY IS BRACING TO COMPENSATE FOR the mind's insecurity. This often presents itself as unnecessary body tension, shallow breathing, constant busyness, the inability to unwind or relax, and "waiting for the other shoe to drop." When these moments arise, pause and identify how your body is moving. Bring in softness and ease to your movement as much as possible. Imagine your body melting or oozing, especially in your upper torso, as you release tension and worry in the present moment and gain a sense of peace and calm.

DAY 282
Take a Pause

IF YOU FIND IT DIFFICULT TO BE STILL, THIS IS A PRACTICE IN FIND-ing moments of steadiness in order to trust that your body and mind can endure stillness. As you are moving through your day, pause by leaning or gently holding onto something in your immediate environ-ment. Try leaning on a kitchen counter, pressing into the wall, or sim-ply holding onto the bathroom sink. Finding moments of steadiness throughout your day teaches your nervous system that it is safe to pause and find quiet and stillness.

DAY 283
Explore the Unknown

IT CAN BE HARD TO TRUST THE PROCESS, ESPECIALLY WHEN THAT process is new or unknown. Draw your attention to something that feels unknown. This can be a new path or direction, place, or activity. This shouldn't be something that conjures up panic, but a small amount of anxiety is okay.

What do I notice in my body as I lean in to the unknown?

....
....
....

What do I need to feel stable in times of uncertainty?

....
....
....

How can my movement support me during this time?

....
....
....

DAY 284
Procrastination

BRING TO MIND THE WORD *PROCRASTINATION*. WHAT IS YOUR RELA-tionship with this word? Do you consider yourself a procrastinator? Do you put things off to the last minute? Perhaps you feel that you do your best work under pressure or on a tight deadline.

Notice how this construct lives in your body. How does your pro-crastinator move? What is it protecting you from? What does it need in order to step aside?

Take a moment to dialogue, either through movement or journal-ing, with this part. What is it teaching you?

....

....

....

....

....

....

....

....

....

....

DAY 285
Let's Get Started

INITIATING MOVEMENT OR ACTION CAN BE CHALLENGING WHEN YOU
are frozen or stuck in your body and mind. Remember this equation.

Movement = Momentum = Initiation

Begin to move your body in small ways. A body in motion will stay
in motion. Movement creates momentum, which enables us to initiate
a task. If you find it hard to "get going," simply begin by shifting your
body, trusting that it will take you where you need to go. This could
also lead to more rest or recuperation. Keep in mind this is not lazi-
ness. Even rest can be productive, especially for a body and mind that
cannot relax or be still.

DAY 286
Perfection

DO YOU STRIVE FOR PERFECTION? PERHAPS YOU FIND IT CHALLENG-
ing to engage in something for fear that it will not be perfect. You may
even find that you sabotage yourself by anticipating that, if you cannot do a task perfectly, it's not worth trying.

Give yourself permission to make a mistake—for example, misspell-
ing a word on social media or wearing mismatched socks. Mistakes
are necessary for learning and growth. The goal isn't to be comfortable making big errors in judgment but to feel safe in knowing that
perfection is not feasible and that the pressure to be perfect may be
keeping you from moving on, realizing a dream, or enjoying the present moment.

DAY 287
Make Space for Trust

BUILDING TRUST IN YOURSELF REQUIRES TIME AND SPACE TO LISTEN and identify your needs, desires, and boundaries. Find time in your day to be with your thoughts and feelings. Notice what comes up for you when you create opportunities to listen and trust that you know what you need.

DAY 288
Your Safe Space

IDENTIFY A PLACE IN YOUR IMMEDIATE ENVIRONMENT THAT SERVES as your safe space. This is a place where you feel most able to relax or connect to the present. This should be a place that supports ease and comfort.

Is it possible for me to be my own safe space?

....
....
....

Is it safe to be with my own body and mind?

....
....
....

DAY 289
Find Your Confi-Dance

YOU MAY FIND IT DIFFICULT TO TRUST YOURSELF, ESPECIALLY WHEN you lack confidence or self-esteem. This most often occurs when others have doubted you or instilled a sense of mistrust in your ability to decide what you need.

Identify three postures that exude or display confidence. String these postures together to form your own dance of confidence. You can choreograph your experience, moving your body in ways that support and encourage self-esteem and ability.

DAY 290
Taking Charge

YOU MAY TAKE A BACKSEAT IN PLANNING OR ORGANIZING SOME-thing because you doubt your ability or fear responsibility. What does it look like to take charge? How would your body express or exude "taking charge"? How difficult is it for you to connect to your ability to be in charge or to manage?

....

....

....

....

....

....

....

....

....

....

....

....

....

....

....

....

....

....

DAY 291
Hope

MAKE A LIST OF ALL THE THINGS YOU COULD HOPE FOR. THEY CAN BE based in reality or fantasy. Reflect on the list and (1) notice where you feel hope in your body and (2) move in a way that instills or supports hope.

....

....

....

....

....

....

....

....

....

....

....

....

....

....

....

....

....

....

....

....

....

....

....

DAY 292
Become Reliable

MAKE PLANS WITH SOMEONE AND KEEP THOSE PLANS. YOU CAN plan to meet up and talk or to do something together. This is an exercise in trusting that you can follow through with your words and intentions.

DAY 293
Promise

HAVE YOU EVER MADE A PROMISE TO YOURSELF? DID YOU BREAK IT? How did it feel when you broke your own promise? Do you trust that you can keep a promise to yourself? What do you need in order to keep a promise?

....
....
....
....
....
....
....
....
....
....

DAY 294
Betrayal

THINK OF A TIME WHEN SOMEONE BETRAYED YOUR TRUST. WHAT DO you notice in your body? Is there avoidance or resistance? Do you have a hard time letting go or moving on?

....
....
....
....
....
....
....
....
....
....
....
....
....
....
....
....
....
....
....
....
....
....

DAY 295
Get Lost

EVEN IF YOU HAVE A COMPROMISED SENSE OF DIRECTION, THERE IS A benefit to getting lost and finding yourself again. This exercise is more about exploring your environment than it is about actually getting lost. Identify an unfamiliar part of your neighborhood or city to explore. When exploring your environment, be sure to identify ways that you can contact someone or make your way back to your starting point or home base. The lesson here is trusting yourself to find your own way or ask for directions. It is not meant to trigger your survival instincts. Feel free to have technology or maps with you for backup.

DAY 296

Building Trust

YOU ARE GOING TO PRACTICE BUILDING TRUST FROM WITHIN BY stacking your spine. Start by sitting or standing in a relaxed position. Notice your current posture. Allow your spine to curve forward as your shoulders slouch and your head droops. Imagine your spine is a zipper. Slowly begin zipping your spine from your tailbone to your head, one vertebra at a time, rolling up until you are lengthened and lifted.

DAY 297
Find Balance . . . Again

THIS IS A TIME TO CHECK IN WITH THE EARLIER EXPERIENCE OF finding your balance (in the section starting with Day 121). Trust that you can bring yourself back to a sense of balance when you notice you are physically or emotionally unsteady. Coming back to center from rocking or swaying, pausing while walking, or catching yourself as you playfully stumble or fall are all ways to support balance.

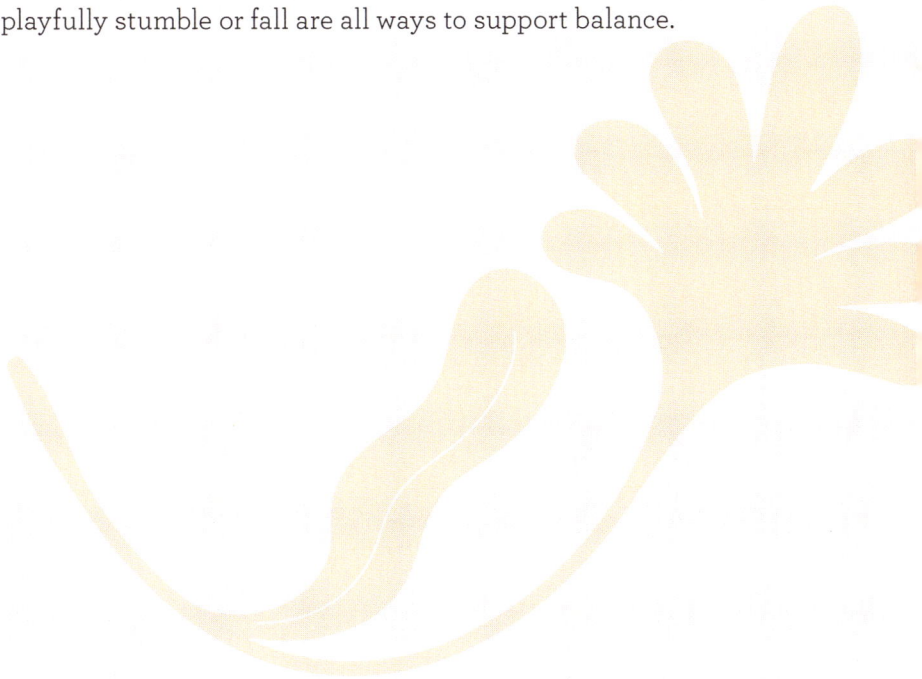

DAY 298
Core Values

You might mistrust yourself when you don't have a solid understanding or grasp of your core values and beliefs. Our core, or torso, holds our value system. Connect to your core values by connecting to your chest, belly, and spine. Find your sense of self as you explore these parts through touch, sensation, and movement.

After this exercise, take five minutes to journal about or list what you consider to be your core values and beliefs.

....
....
....
....
....
....
....
....
....
....

DAY 299
Got Your Back

YOU MAY HAVE EXPERIENCE IN "HAVING SOMEONE'S BACK," BUT DO you have your own? Take five minutes to explore and connect with your back space, such as through touch, support, or moving from the back of the body (for instance, walking backward).

What do you notice about your sensation of trust as you move through this exploration?

....

....

....

....

....

....

....

....

....

....

DAY 300
How Are You *Moving?*

REFLECT ON YOUR EXPERIENCE AND CURRENT CONNECTION WITH
trust. Do you trust your own ability to identify and express what you
need? How does trust play a role in your health journey?

....
....
....
....
....
....
....
....
....
....
....
....
....
....
....
....
....
....
....
....

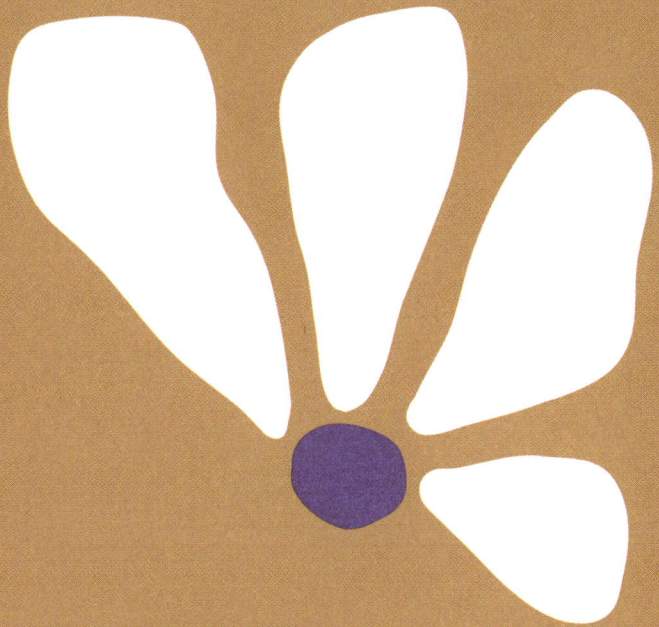

RELATIONSHIPS
AND
ATTACHMENTS

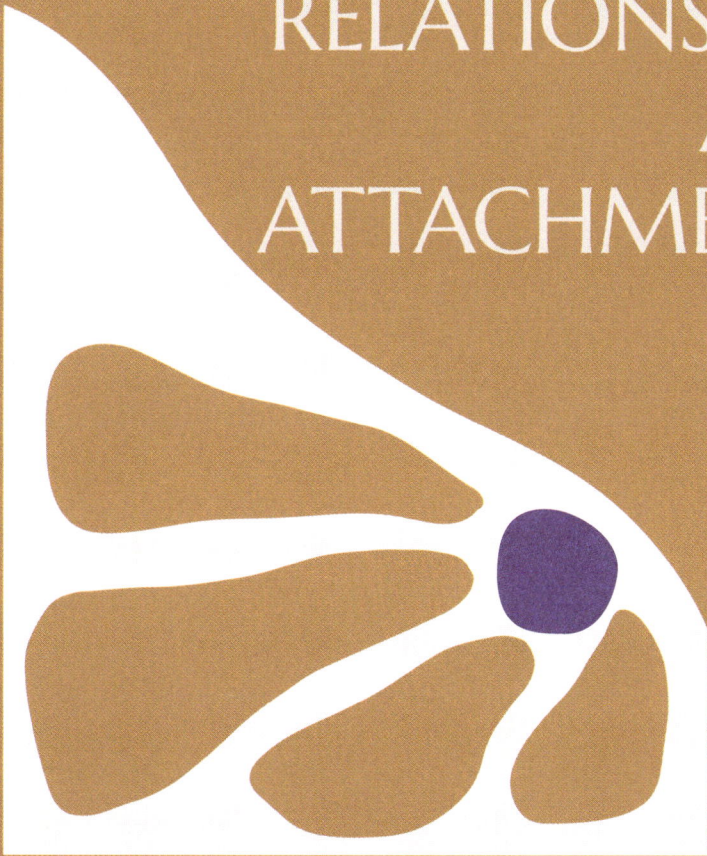

The relationships you have with other bodies is a direct reflection of the one you have with your own.

DAY 301
Your Relationships

REFLECT ON THE CURRENT RELATIONSHIPS IN YOUR LIFE (PEOPLE, places, things, actions) and journal about them.

Next, reflect on the relationships you do not have or the ones you'd like to prioritize.

How do you physically feel about relationships? What sensations and which parts of your body are activated during your reflection?

....

....

....

....

....

....

....

....

....

....

DAY 302
Attached

WHAT DOES IT MEAN TO YOU TO BE ATTACHED? WHOM OR WHAT ARE you attached to? What would you find it difficult to live without? Once you identify an object, bring it close to you. What physical sensations arise in your body that suggest attachment?

....

....

....

....

....

....

....

....

....

....

DAY 303
Find Your Rhythm

IDENTIFY YOUR RHYTHM OF RELATIONSHIP. WHAT DO YOU NOTICE about your past relationships? How do you engage with and disengage from a relationship? Below, draw a pattern reflecting what the rhythm of relationship looks like. Is it smooth, bumpy, severed, winding, or a roller coaster? After you draw the pattern, try moving the pattern with your body and become aware of what your body encounters when in a relationship.

DAY 304
Grudges

WHAT DOES IT FEEL LIKE TO HOLD A GRUDGE? IS THIS SOMETHING you are familiar with? Perhaps you have someone close to you who holds grudges. Notice the qualities of this behavior and reflect on how it feels to hold your grudge.

....

....

....

....

....

....

....

....

....

....

DAY 305
Leaving

YOU MAY FIND THAT LEAVING A RELATIONSHIP IS DIFFICULT OR THAT you want to be the first one to leave so as not to be left behind. Become aware of how you feel when someone leaves before you or how it feels to be the first to leave. Try leaving others at a dinner table to use the restroom, only to return when you are done. You can try this at a party, work meeting, or informal social gathering. Play with being the last one to leave and the first one to leave. This exercise takes more than once to try it out. Here are some questions to reflect on:

Which feels more familiar?

....

....

....

Which is more difficult?

....

....

....

What am I afraid will happen in either scenario?

....

....

....

DAY 306
Lose It

RELATIONSHIPS AND ATTACHMENTS ARE CHALLENGING BECAUSE they often involve loss or fear of losing someone or something. You may find that you avoid attachments to save yourself from feeling grief or loss.

Identify an object that you are attached to and that you access on a semiregular basis. Some examples might be technology, a piece of jewelry, a certain food or beverage, or a hygiene or beauty product. Find a safe place for this object and put it out of sight for twenty-four hours. Reflect on the following questions:

Was I able to go without this object for twenty-four hours?

....
....
....

What was the hardest part of not having access to this object?

....
....
....

What did I find myself doing to cope with the absence?

....
....
....

How did it feel in my body and mind not to have this object?

....
....
....

DAY 307
Let It Go!

NEXT TIME YOU USE THE BATHROOM, PRACTICE PHYSICALLY LETTING go. Relax as much of your body as possible, take a deep cleansing breath, and unclench as you relieve yourself. Additionally, you can bring to mind something you want to let go of emotionally to support a sense of grounding, relaxation, and stability.

DAY 308
Transitional Object

THINK BACK TO WHEN YOU WERE A YOUNG CHILD. PERHAPS YOU HAD a pacifier, blanket, or stuffed animal that helped soothe you. These are often known as *transitional objects*, objects that allow you to feel secure and connected when your caregivers leave. Identify an object, soft blanket, pillow, stuffed animal, or even a piece of fabric that you can use as a transitional object to find comfort and stability in the absence of someone. How does it feel to have this "security blanket" of sorts? Become aware of how your body moves in the presence of security.

DAY 309
Secure

THE OPTIMAL ATTACHMENT IS A SECURE ATTACHMENT. TAKE A moment to bring the idea of security into your body. How does secure move? When do you feel this in your life?

....

....

....

....

....

....

....

....

....

....

DAY 310
Flags

WHAT ARE YOUR RED FLAGS IN A RELATIONSHIP? WHAT DOES A RED flag feel like in your body? What sensations does it create? Where did you learn these? Are they productive or protective?

....

....

....

....

Now consider what your green flags are in a relationship. What does a green flag look like in your body? How did you learn these?

....

....

....

....

How useful are these flags when it comes to creating a secure relationship with someone?

....

....

....

....

DAY 311
Love Scoops

DR. KATHLYN HENDRICKS, AUTHOR, DANCE/MOVEMENT THERAPIST, and somatic coach, talks about "fear melters," powerful moves designed to shift us from states of fear to states of flow. "Love scoops" are a beautiful exercise in bringing love, attention, and affection toward yourself. Begin with your feet firmly planted on the floor and your knees softly bent. Allow your arms together or individually to scoop down and around as you bring love into your heart space. Feel the love you want to receive.

Is it difficult for me to receive love?

....

....

....

....

In what ways does my body limit, restrict, or close itself off to love?

....

....

....

....

DAY 312
Attention!

EVERYONE WANTS AND NEEDS ATTENTION. IF YOUR BODY DOESN'T receive it, your mind will crave it. Take a moment to embody *attention*. How does attention move? Consider the different constructs of attention, such as *paying attention, calling to one's attention, attention seeking, giving or receiving attention*, and *standing at attention*.

Reflect on the qualities of attention as you feel it move your body.

DAY 313
Affection

THINK OF THE WAYS IN WHICH YOU SHOW AFFECTION AND THE WAYS you want to be shown affection. Are they similar or different? What happens when you do not receive affection, especially in the ways you want? Do you increase your outward affection or withhold it when it is not reciprocated?

DAY 314
Nurture a Neutral Part

IDENTIFY A PART OF YOUR BODY THAT YOU FEEL NEUTRAL TOWARD. You don't have any judgment one way or the other for this part. Once you have identified it and brought it into your awareness, find a way to console, support, and nurture this body part. How would this part like to be touched or acknowledged? Is it difficult to connect to this part? How does this part feel about being nurtured?

....

....

....

....

....

....

....

....

....

....

DAY 315
Nurture a Neglected Body Part

IDENTIFY A PART OF YOUR BODY THAT YOU HAVE NEGLECTED OR ignored. Once you have identified it and brought it into your awareness, find a way to console, support, and nurture this body part. How would this part like to be touched or acknowledged? Is it difficult to connect to this part? How does this part feel about being nurtured?

....

....

....

....

....

....

....

....

....

DAY 316
Sparking Connection

GO THROUGH YOUR BELONGINGS AND IDENTIFY THINGS THAT YOU feel a connection to. Notice the stories you tell yourself about these items. Do these narratives feel supportive and inviting, or do they feel like an excuse to cling to a past version of yourself?

DAY 317
Parting Ways

PART WAYS WITH AN ITEM THAT NO LONGER SERVES YOU, SUCH AS A piece of clothing, furniture, or household accessory. Notice the emotional attachment you have to this item. Can you see this object for what it is versus how it makes you feel?

....

....

....

....

....

....

....

....

....

....

DAY 318
Make Yourself a Priority

LEARNING TO BE WITH YOURSELF IS A VALUABLE SKILL. MAKE PLANS with yourself and keep them. Prioritize what you want and how you want to be treated. Journal on what this experience was like for you.

....

....

....

....

....

....

....

....

....

....

....

DAY 319
Coregulate with Nature

HEALTHY RELATIONSHIPS INVOLVE COREGULATION. IF YOU DO NOT have someone to regulate with, you can regulate with Mother Nature. Some ideas: sway with the breeze, shake with the leaves, walk barefoot in the grass, and feel the warmth of the sun on your face.

DAY 320
Deepen Your Relationship with Nature

REFLECT ON THE PREVIOUS EXERCISE, AND THEN FIND AN OPPORTU-nity to relate with the things around you—for example, the sound of the birds, the temperature of the air, the shape of the clouds. What elements of nature provide comfort and support during a busy day?

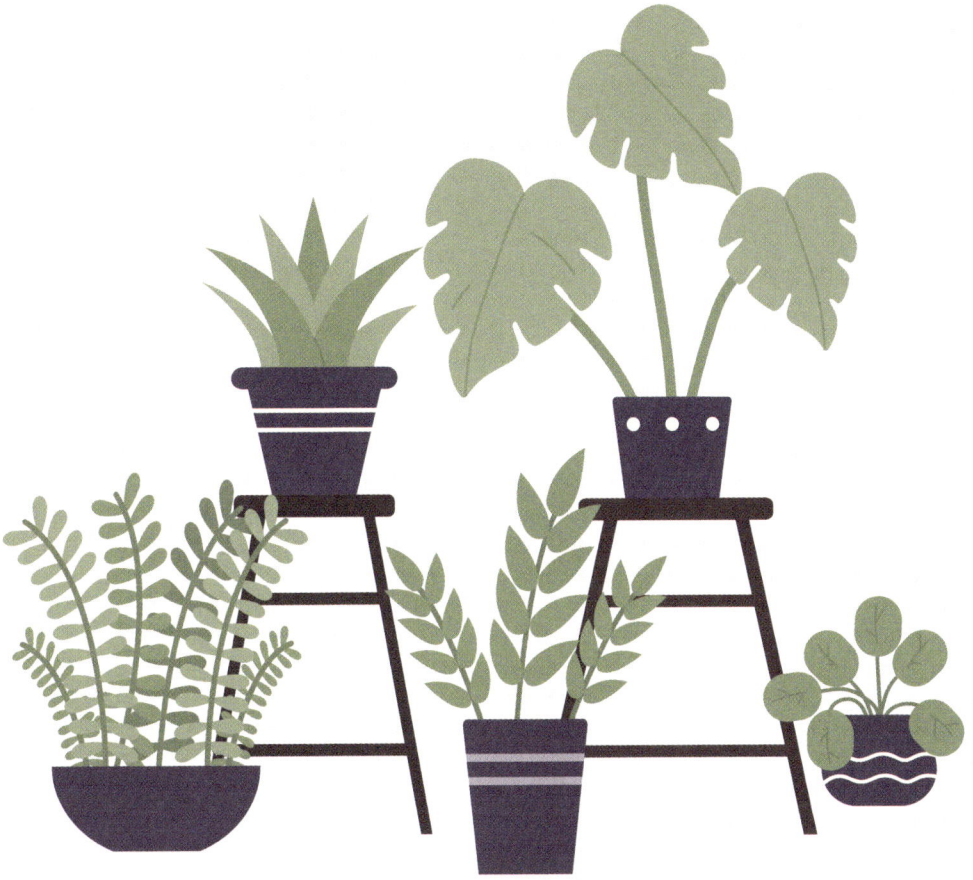

DAY 321
Take Care

ALLOW YOURSELF TO CARE FOR SOMETHING THAT DOESN'T PLACE
conditions on you. Water someone's plants or take care of a pet.

DAY 322
Back-to-Back

Sit back-to-back with someone you respect and trust. Allow each other to provide an even amount of support. Try to match your breathing patterns. Talk about how this feels together.

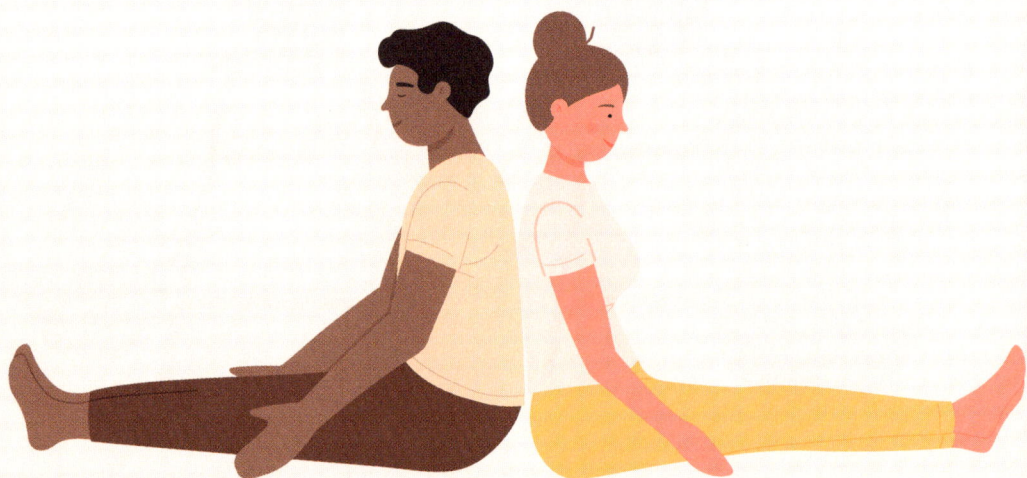

DAY 323
Prioritize an Existing Relationship

MAKE TIME TO BE WITH A FRIEND, SIGNIFICANT OTHER, OR FAMILY member. What do you value most about this relationship? Tell the person.

DAY 324
Make a New Friend

FRIENDSHIP IS NECESSARY AT ALL AGES, AND OFTEN IT IS HARDER TO make new friends as we get older. Although it takes time to build a friendship, this prompt is an exercise in prioritizing this need. Make an effort to reach out to someone new. Notice how it feels in your body to engage in this exercise. Become aware of the emotions that arise as you open yourself to the possibility of a new relationship.

DAY 325
Find Pleasure

MAKE A LIST OF THINGS THAT BRING YOU PLEASURE. ENGAGE IN TWO
or three things on this list. How do you identify pleasure in your body?
Where do you feel it most? On the contrary, how does your body move
in the absence of pleasure?

....

....

....

....

....

....

....

DAY 326
Connect Through Body Language

REVISIT THE PROMPT FROM DAY 164. TRY MATCHING SOMEONE'S body language while in conversation. Take this opportunity to feel what it is like to move in someone else's shoes. This can be through posture or gesture. How does this feel for you? Do you notice anything in the other person following this exercise? What does this do for your relationship?

....

....

....

....

....

....

....

....

....

....

....

DAY 327
Embrace Yourself

Give yourself a hug.

DAY 328

Connect to Your Body

Make the relationship you have with your body a priority throughout the day. Connect to the physical sensations present. Move your body in ways that feel supportive, nurturing, and rejuvenating.

DAY 329
Offer Assistance

CONNECT WITH SOMEONE, A FRIEND OR STRANGER, IN NEED. REMEMber to listen to your body for cues of safety and healthy boundaries. It is vital that you honor your own needs and boundaries when supporting someone else rather than neglect or override them. Ideally, take action through movement, not just a monetary donation.

Journal on this experience, reflecting on what you noticed about your and the other person's body language and nonverbal communication. Was it difficult to support someone else? How does your body feel in relation to someone in need? What does it feel like to ask for help and receive it?

DAY 330
How Are You *Moving?*

WHAT AWARENESS HAVE YOU BUILT AROUND YOUR BODY AND RELA-
tionship and attachment? How might your perspective on relationship and attachment change going forward?

....

....

....

....

....

....

....

....

....

....

....

....

....

....

....

....

....

....

....

....

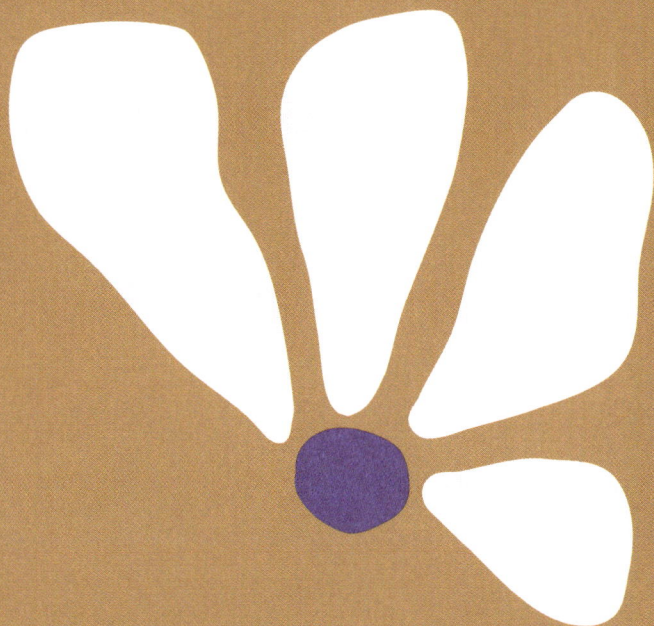

MOVING
EMOTIONS

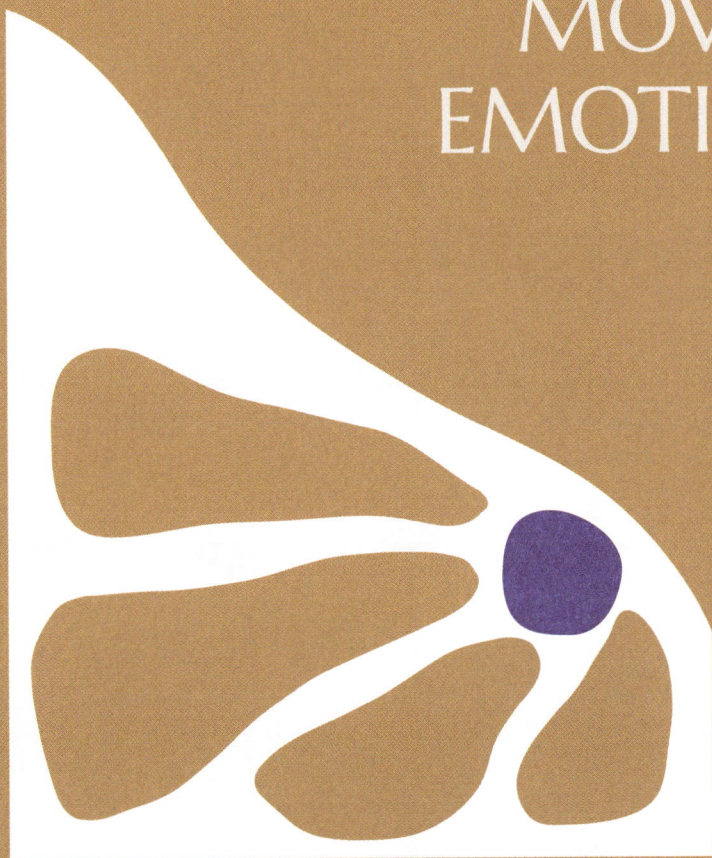

Freedom from an emotion
doesn't come from letting it go
but rather from letting it in.

DAY 331
Common Emotions

MAKE A LIST OF COMMON EMOTIONS YOU ENCOUNTER IN YOURSELF.
Under each emotion, list when you feel it (time of day or year, circumstance, environment, or situation). Don't try to find logic or reason or
try so much to answer why you feel what you feel. Notice the when
and the how of the emotion.

1. ....

2. ....

3. ....

4. ....

5. ....

6. ....

7. ....

DAY 332
Heel Rock

LIE DOWN ON A FIRM SURFACE AND REMOVE YOUR SHOES. RELAX your arms, hands palms down, at your sides. Begin gently rocking your heels, softly flexing your toes toward the ceiling. Allow this movement to create flow between your feet, pelvis, chest, and jaw. The absence of flow in the body signals where emotions might be stuck. Adjust your body as needed to support relaxation and release of tension. Remember to breathe to support your movement.

DAY 333

Stuck

FEELING STUCK IN YOUR MIND AND BODY? BECOME AWARE OF HOW you are stuck in your body and make small shifts to your posture. Keep shifting until you feel your body move through the "stuckness."

DAY 334
Express a Feeling

IDENTIFY A FEELING IN THE PRESENT MOMENT AND EXPRESS IT through movement. Here are some ideas:

Anger = *stomp your feet*
Joy = *jump*
Anxiety = *shake or bounce*

These are just a few examples. Only you know what your body needs. Listen to it and express your emotion in a way that feels authentic to you.

DAY 335
Expand to Express

MOVING THROUGH AN EMOTION MENTALLY REQUIRES SPACE FOR THE emotion to move physically. Bring awareness to the current space your body is taking up and find a way to expand it. Spread your body out in any way that feels possible to create more internal capacity.

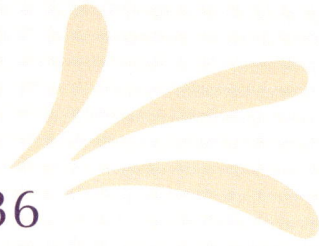

DAY 336
Familiar Versus Unfamiliar Emotions

MAKE A LIST OF EMOTIONS THAT YOU ARE FAMILIAR WITH AND A list of emotions that you are not so familiar with. This doesn't mean positive or negative but rather the emotions that you allow yourself to express or feel versus the ones you suppress or try to hide.

familiar

....

....

....

....

....

....

....

....

....

....

unfamiliar

....

....

....

....

....

....

....

....

....

....

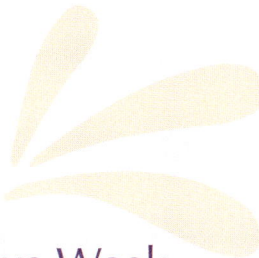

DAY 337
Strong Versus Weak

Take an inventory of the emotions that you qualify as strong emotions and the ones you qualify as weak emotions. Do you agree with your list? Is there a benefit to calling an emotion strong versus weak? How do you feel physically toward the weak emotions?

strong

weak

....
....
....
....
....
....
....
....
....
....

DAY 338
Range of Motion

YOUR RANGE OF EMOTION IS INFLUENCED BY YOUR RANGE OF MOTION. Revisit the earlier section on mobilization (starting at Day 91) and find ways to mobilize your body to support a greater range of motion. Reflect on how mobilizing your body influences your mood and emotional landscape.

DAY 339
Expressive Movement

MOVE OR WALK IN A WAY THAT EXPRESSES YOUR CURRENT MOOD.

DAY 340
Moving Judgment

RECALL A TIME THAT YOU FELT JUDGED. NOTICE HOW YOUR BODY moves. Reflect on what happens to your movement when you feel the judgment of others.

DAY 341

Move How You Want to Feel

MOVE OR WALK IN A WAY THAT SUPPORTS HOW YOU WOULD LIKE TO feel. Embrace movements and qualities of movement that facilitate the emotion you wish to experience. For example, if you wish to feel happier, engage in movements that you associate with happiness.

DAY 342
Emotional Efficiency

LOCATE TWO POINTS IN YOUR HOME OR CURRENT ENVIRONMENT that are at least ten feet apart. Label one point A and the other point B. Starting at point A, move as efficiently as possible to point B. And return to point A. Next, move from point A to point B as inefficiently as possible. And return to point A.

What did I notice between the two exercises?

....
....
....

Which is more familiar to me?

....
....
....

What was the most challenging part?

....

....

....

What surprised me the most?

....

....

....

What insights does this provide into how I move through my emotions?

....

....

....

DAY 343
Emotion Mapping

PRINT OR DRAW A BLANK FIGURE OF A PERSON. NEXT, IDENTIFY TWO or three emotions that are readily available to you or that feel most familiar. Choose a color (marker or pen) that represents each emotion. Create a map key similar to this one but using your own emotions. Add a design, line, or image that represents what this emotion looks like.

MAP KEY

★ ★ ★ = Happy   ♥ ♥ ♥ = Love

●●● = Sad   XXX = Anxiety

||||||| = Angry   OOO = Surprised

Bring to mind one emotion and a circumstance when you felt that way. On a scale of 1 to 10, think of a situation that conjures up a 3 or a 4 in terms of intensity. Become aware of where you feel this emotion in your body and identify it on your figure. Be as specific as possible. Repeat this process with the other emotions.

Then, reflect on the following questions:

Which parts of the figure stand out to me?

....

....

Which parts have been left blank?

....

....

Am I surprised by anything I see on the figure?

....

....

DAY 344
Dance It Out

Become aware of an emotion you are currently feeling. Find a song that represents that emotion for you, through its lyrics, rhythm, or instrumentation. Allow yourself to move to and be moved by the song. This is another way to express and move an emotion that you are experiencing rather than simply verbalizing it.

DAY 345
DANCE Party

To dance is to

Dispel
Anxious
Nervous
Constricted
Energy

Have an impromptu DANCE party in your home, car, or office. Give yourself a few minutes to release the tension or friction in your body.

DAY 346
ACE Your Mental Health

BECOME **A**WARE OF HOW YOUR BODY IS HOLDING A CURRENT FEELing or emotion.

CHALLENGE the way your body is moving in this emotion.

EXPRESS this emotion through more movement.

DAY 347
Move Your Age

SOMETIMES, WHEN WE ARE TRIGGERED, WE REVERT BACK TO THE AGE at which the initial trauma occurred. In those moments, we can move toward movement that is more in line with our current age.

Bring to mind a situation when you felt activated, triggered, or overwhelmed. Ask yourself, *How old do I feel?* Notice the mannerisms, posture, and movements associated with this "age." How do they support the age you identified? How might you be able to shift or challenge them in order to move as your current age?

....

....

....

....

....

....

....

DAY 348
Where Do I Feel My . . . ?

NEXT TIME YOU BECOME AWARE OF AN INTENSE EMOTION, ASK YOUR-self the following questions:

Where do I feel it?

....

....

....

How do I know I feel this way?

....

....

....

If I couldn't use my words, how would others know I feel this way?

....

....

....

DAY 349
Body (Part) Talk

IDENTIFY A PART OF YOUR BODY WHERE YOU FEEL TENSION OR FRIC-
tion. Ask yourself, *If this part could talk, what might it say?* Put words
to what this part is feeling. What does it want you to know?

....

....

....

....

....

....

....

....

....

....

....

....

....

....

....

....

....

....

....

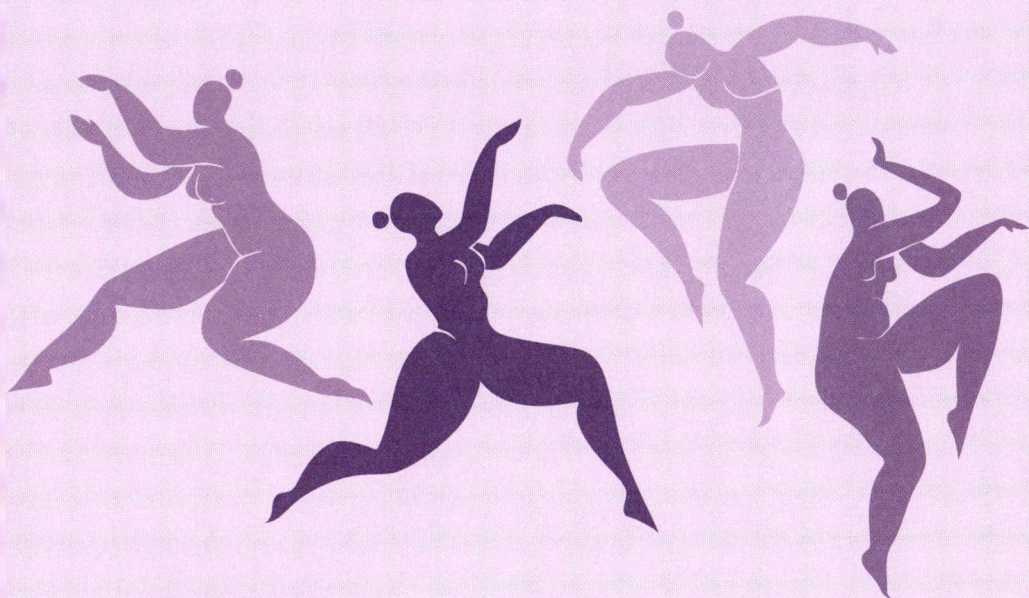

DAY 350
The Dance of . . .

IDENTIFY FIVE EMOTIONS THAT YOU EXPERIENCE THE MOST. CREATE an impromptu dance of each emotion. Notice the different qualities of each emotion. Which ones have similarities, and which ones feel different?

DAY 351
Move Your Seat

YOUR HIPS HOLD SO MUCH OF YOUR EMOTIONAL EXPERIENCES. SPEND three to five minutes moving your hips. Shake, wiggle, or roll them to release stored emotional tension.

DAY 352

Resistance

THROUGH THIS PROCESS, YOU MAY HAVE EXPERIENCED SOME HESItancy or resistance to feeling, processing, or simply acknowledging an emotion. Take a moment to identify where in your body you hold resistance. How does it show up in these places? Lean in to the resistance.

What do you need to accept what you feel? Keep in mind that resistance is a means of protection. This is a good time to revisit movements that support stability and regulation to feel secure in yourself when faced with a perceived threat to your emotional safety.

....

....

....

....

....

....

....

....

DAY 353
On the Defense

DEFENSIVENESS IS PROTECTING YOURSELF FROM YOUR FEELINGS OF hurt or shame. Defensiveness might protect your self-esteem, but it can harm your relationships. Imagine you are the defense player on a team who is trying to stop the offense from scoring a point. What does it feel like in your body to defend? What postures, gestures, or movements do you notice? Intentionally shift into a position of receptivity and curiosity. What happens to your defensiveness when you are open to feedback?

....

....

....

....

....

....

....

....

....

....

DAY 354
Avoidance

BRING TO MIND ALL THE WAYS YOU AVOID YOUR FEELINGS. WHAT habits or activities do you rely on to avoid emotional discomfort or pain? Try to identify where and when this behavior began.

....

....

....

....

....

....

....

....

....

....

DAY 355
Feeling Narratives

BECOME AWARE OF WHAT YOU SEE AROUND YOU AS YOU MOVE through your day. Name emotions as you see them in the world, not just as you experience them yourself. Which emotions do you see others display as you observe from a distance? What suggests this emotion to you? In which ways is their body talking that reinforces the emotion(s) you see?

....

....

....

....

....

....

....

....

....

....

DAY 356
Shift Your Mood

MOVE YOUR BODY TO MOVE YOUR MIND. IF YOU ARE EXPERIENCING an intense emotion or a less-than-favorable mood, get moving. There is no right way to do it. Move in any way possible no matter how small or slow.

DAY 357

Shift Your Perspective

MOVE TO A NEW LOCATION IN THE ROOM TO SEE A NEW PERSPECTIVE. Notice what calls your attention or notice something you never noticed before.

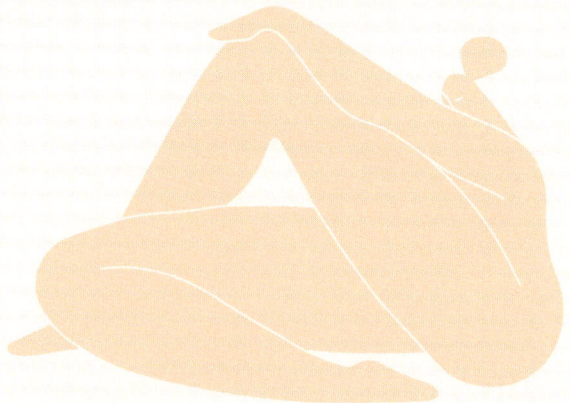

DAY 358
Make Time for Emotions

SPEND TIME DOING AN ACTIVITY THAT EVOKES AN EMOTION YOU want to feel more of. Watch a movie that moves you to tears or laughter. Take a dance class. Try out martial arts. Paint or write. Make time for the emotions that you want to feel more of.

DAY 359
Stomp and Shout, Let It Out!

ANY TIME YOU FEEL OVERWHELMED OR ACTIVATED BY AN INTENSE emotion, allow yourself to stomp or shout (not at someone) to diffuse the intensity.

DAY 360
Movement Check-In

CONNECTION TO YOUR BODY ISN'T ABOUT ADDING MOVEMENT BUT about looking at the movement that is already present.

Identify all the ways your body is moving in this moment and write them down.

....
....
....
....
....
....
....
....
....
....
....
....
....
....
....
....
....
....
....
....

DAY 361
Know Your Worth

YOU ARE NOT WORTHY BECAUSE OF WHAT YOUR body can do but simply because it exists. Honor all the ways you exist and take up space in this world.

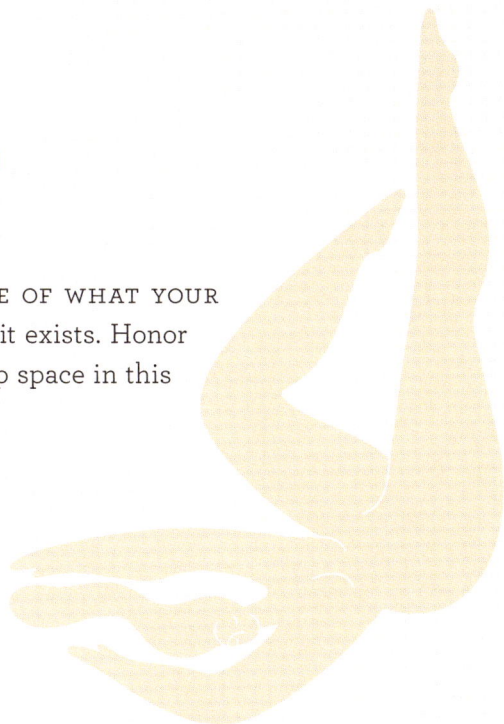

DAY 362

Dance Like Everyone Is Watching

DANCE IS EXPRESSION OF THE SELF; THEREFORE, AVOIDING IT ISN'T self-preservation but rather self-denial. Dance is rhythmic body movement that expresses a thought or idea. Commit to dancing a few minutes every day!

DAY 363
Think and Feel

FEELING BETTER STARTS WITH FEELING. YOU CANNOT REGULATE emotions you don't feel.

This is your reminder to make space for feeling, not just thinking.

DAY 364
Thank Your Body

FIND A WAY TO THANK YOUR BODY FOR ALL IT HAS DONE OVER THE past 364 days—all the ways it kept you safe, supported, grounded, aware, and responsive. Your body is an incredible thing, as are you! Take time to celebrate all your body is capable of.

DAY 365
How Are You *Moving* Today?

IDENTIFY THE WAYS YOUR MIND AND BODY FELT SUPPORTED IN MOV-
ing through your emotions over the last thirty days. Write down all
the ways that you will continue to support moving through your
emotions.

....

....

....

....

....

....

....

....

....

....

....

....

....

....

....

....

....

....

....

DAY 366
Leap Year Bonus

Leap!

Play leapfrog.

Leap for joy!

Use this extra day as an opportunity to expand your movement repertoire and incorporate elements of leaping into your day.

Additional Resources

Caldwell, Christine. *Conscious Moving: An Embodied Guide for Healing, Learning, Contemplating, and Creating.* North Atlantic Books, 2024.

Caldwell, Christine, and David I. Rome. *Bodyfulness: Somatic Practices for Presence, Empowerment, and Waking Up in This Life.* Shambhala, 2018.

Kennedy, R. *Anxiety Rx: A Revolutionary New Prescription for Anxiety Relief—from the Doctor Who Created It.* St. Martin's Essentials, 2024.

Mann, Jennifer, and Karden Rabin. *The Secret Language of the Body: Regulate Your Nervous System, Heal Your Body, Free Your Mind.* HarperOne, 2024.

Marich, Jamie, and Christine Valters Paintner. *Dancing Mindfulness: A Creative Path to Healing and Transformation.* SkyLight Paths, 2016.

Van der Kolk, Bessel A. *The Body Keeps the Score: Mind, Brain and Body in the Transformation of Trauma.* Penguin Books, 2015.

Acknowledgments

I WANT TO THANK EVERYONE WHO HELD AND WHO CONTINUES TO hold space for me to experience my body and to challenge the thoughts in my mind. A special shout out to Nikki Levine, Kimberly Romic, and Stacy Goldman, who continue to hold space for and teach me healthy ways to come home to my body.

Thank you to my clients, who allow me to practice being in my body while simultaneously connecting to someone else's every day.

Thank you to my agent, Linda Konner, for continuing to support my projects and find amazing homes for them. Thank you to Nana K. Twumasi and the entire Balance team for creating a warm and welcoming home for *BodyTalk*.

Thank you to my family, who loves me for who I am and not just what I think.

Last, thank you to my body, for carrying me through this life and continuing to talk even when I forget to listen.

About the Author

ERICA HORNTHAL, LCPC, BC-DMT, IS AN INTERNATIONALLY renowned board-certified dance/movement therapist, licensed clinical professional counselor, and author with a thriving practice supporting individuals all over the world on a journey to rediscover their mind–body connection. Erica's area of expertise has caught the attention of multiple publications, including The *New York Times*, *Epoch Times*, *Dance Magazine*, *Reader's Digest*, and *PARADE*. She is the author of the "Body Awareness for Mental Health" course, *Body Aware: Rediscover Your Mind–Body Connection, Stop Feeling Stuck, and Improve Your Mental Health with Simple Movement Practices*, and *The Movement Therapy Card Deck: 52 Mindful Movement Exercises to Regulate Your Nervous System and Process Trauma*. Erica has built a following that embraces the power of movement for mental health.